The Moringa Tree

What you don't know can heal you!

I0429490

Joe Urbach
www.gardeningaustin.com
www.phytonutrientfarms.com

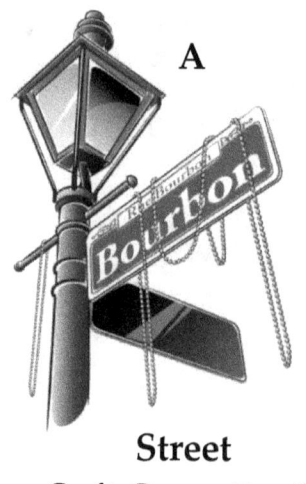

A

Street
Soft Cover Book

1st published in the United State in 2016 by
Bond Street Publications, a Hojo Enterprises Company

1st Printing 2016

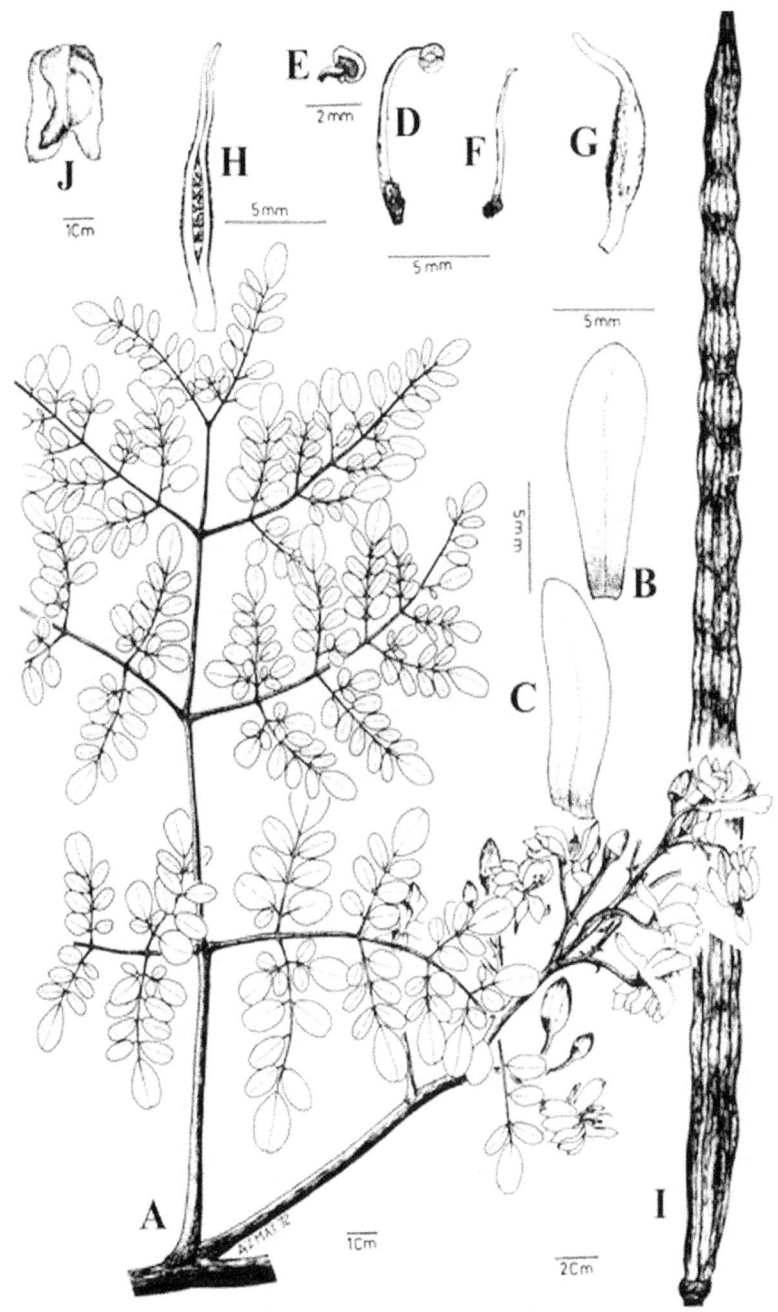

Moringa oleifera: A, Branch; B, Petal; C, Sepal; D, Fertile stamen; E, Anthers; F, Sterile stamen; G, Carpel; H, L.S. of ovary; I, Fruit; J, Seed.

Nutrient Chart

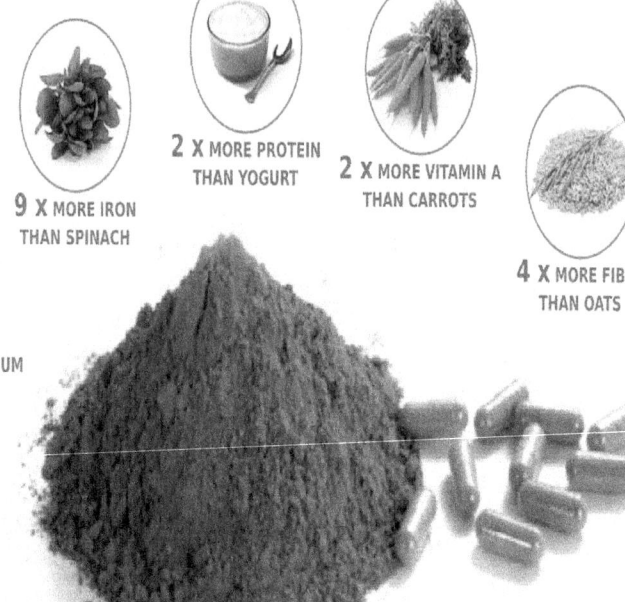

9 X MORE IRON
THAN SPINACH

2 X MORE PROTEIN
THAN YOGURT

2 X MORE VITAMIN A
THAN CARROTS

4 X MORE FIBER
THAN OATS

4 X MORE POTASSIUM
THAN BANANAS

14 X MORE CALCIUM
THAN MILK

Gram per Gram comparison *

Some antioxidants present in Moringa

Alanine	Delta 7-Avenasterol	Prolamine
Alpha-Carotene	Glutathione	Proline
Arginine	Histidine	Quercetin
Beta-Carotene	Indole Acetic Acid	Rutin
Beta-Sitosterol	Indoleacetonitrile	Selenium
Caffeoylquinic Acid	Kaempferal	Threonine
Campesterol	Leucine	Tryptophan
Carotenoids	Lutein	Xanthins
Chlorophyll	Methionine	Xanthophyll
Chromium	Myristic Acid	Zeatin
Delta 5-Avenasterol	Palmitic Acid	Zeaxanthin

Vitamins

Vitamin A (Carotene)
Vitamin B1 (Thiamin)
Vitamin B2 (Riboflavin)
Vitamin B3 (Niacin)
Vitamin B6 (Pyridoxine)
Vitamin B7 (Biotin)
Vitamin C
Vitamin D
Vitamin E
Vitamin K

Minerals

Alpha-Carotene	Proline
Arginine	Quercetin
Beta-Carotene	Rutin
Beta-Sitosterol	Selenium
Caffeoylquinic Acid	Threonine
Campesterol	Tryptophan
Glutathione	Indoleacetonitrile
Histidine	Kaempferal
Indole Acetic Acid	Leucine

Essential Amino Acids

Phenylalanine	Tryptophan	Isoleucine	Lysine
Threonine	Valine	Leucine	Methionine

Non-essential Amino Acids

Alanine	Aspartic Acid	Glutamine	Histidine	Serine
Arginine	Cystine	Glycine	Proline	Tyrosine

DEDICATION

This book is for my very good friend Mr. Robbie Warner. That's him →

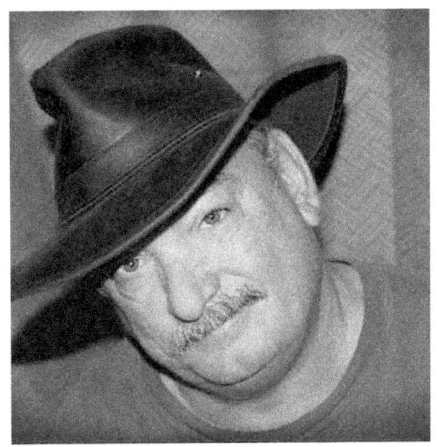

I had the privilege of introducing Robbie to the Moringa Tree and though he does not know it, a brief comment he made about Moringa led to this book.

Basically he said,
> *"I looked online and there is a ton of stuff on Moringa, but it is all anecdotal, where is the science, brother, where is the science?"*

I hope, my friend, that I have included enough science in this work for you!

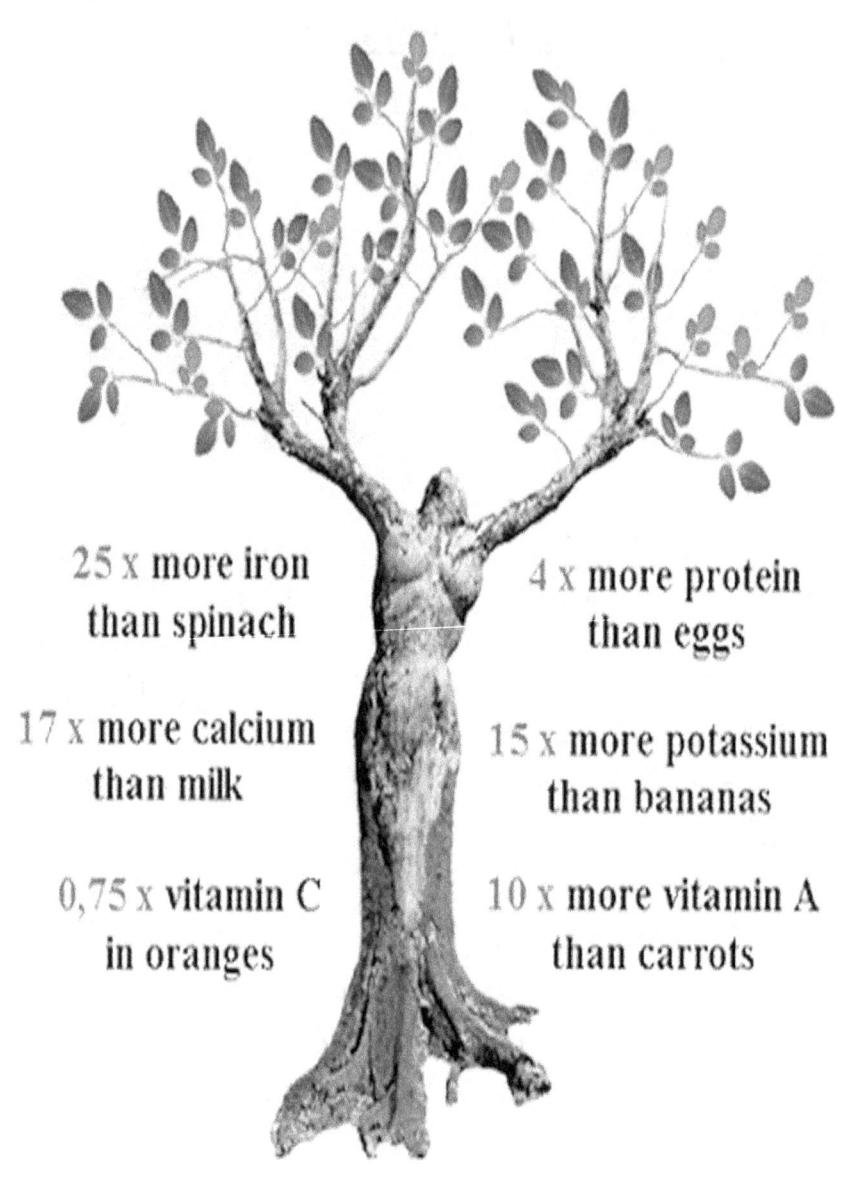

Table of Contents

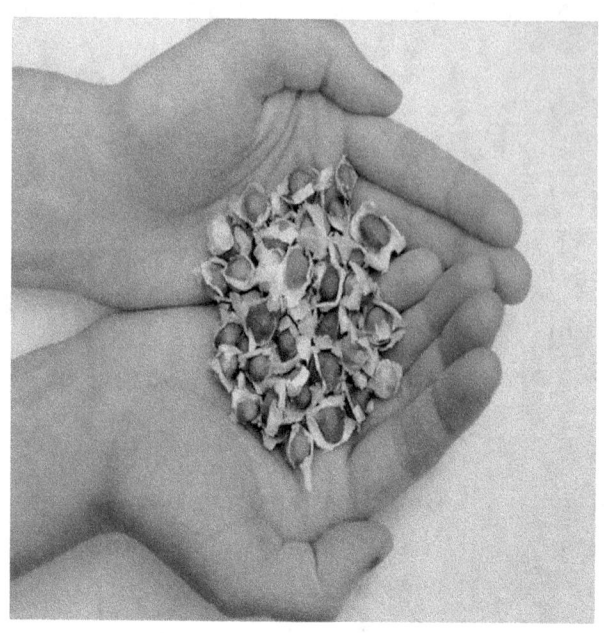

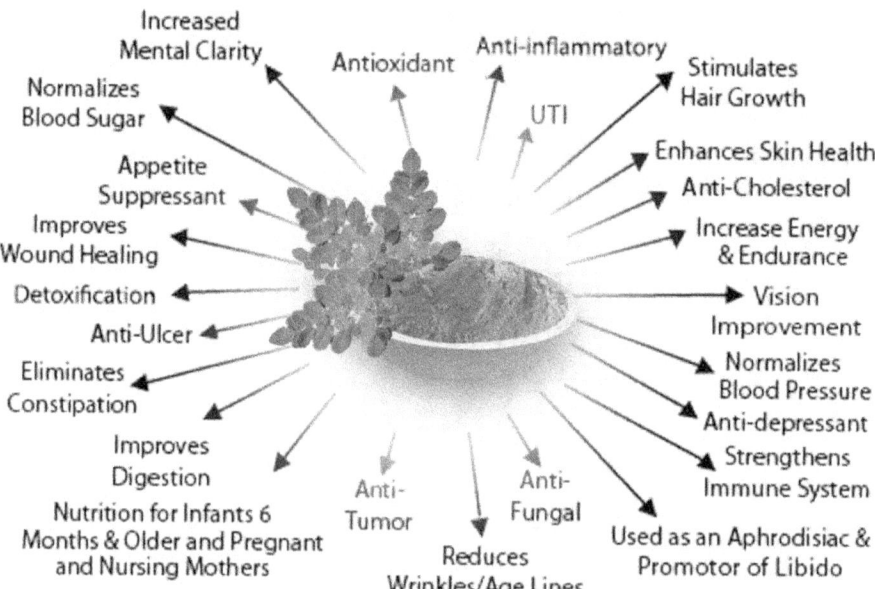

Increased
Mental Clarity

Antioxidant

Anti-inflammatory

Stimulates
Hair Growth

Normalizes
Blood Sugar

UTI

Appetite
Suppressant

Enhances Skin Health

Anti-Cholesterol

Improves
Wound Healing

Increase Energy
& Endurance

Detoxification

Vision
Improvement

Anti-Ulcer

Normalizes
Blood Pressure

Eliminates
Constipation

Anti-depressant

Strengthens
Immune System

Improves
Digestion

Anti-
Tumor

Anti-
Fungal

Nutrition for Infants 6
Months & Older and Pregnant
and Nursing Mothers

Reduces
Wrinkles/Age Lines

Used as an Aphrodisiac &
Promotor of Libido

Forward

I am not a scientist, nor a medical doctor, nor a nutritionist nor any other kind of healthcare worker. I am not a research professional nor have I ever been involved in research or any kind.

I am a gardener, a father, a grandfather, and a diabetic. All of this led me to my concern about nutrition, and in turn, led me on a quest that eventually led to the writing of this book. My journey of exploration has convinced me that there is a very serious problem with the fruit and vegetables that are finding their way into our local markets and eventually on to our dinner plates. The real concern is that it soon can impact our health. In addition, half of the children on planet Earth live in poverty conditions, many suffering malnutrition and forced to drink polluted or tainted water. In this day and age, with all the modern advances of man, this situation is completely unacceptable.

The information I present in this work is provided for your consideration only and I absolutely do not condone, endorse, or recommend that you change any of your diet or exercise habits without first consulting your healthcare professional.

My belief is that knowledge is power and my goal is to empower you with the information that follows so that you and your doctor can choose the best course of action for you to take to help you achieve a better, healthier, happier, and longer life!

I Am Not A Doctor

The information presented here is accurate to the best of my knowledge.

I am not a doctor therefore this information is not intended to diagnose, treat, cure or prevent any disease because only doctors can do that.

Please do your own research!

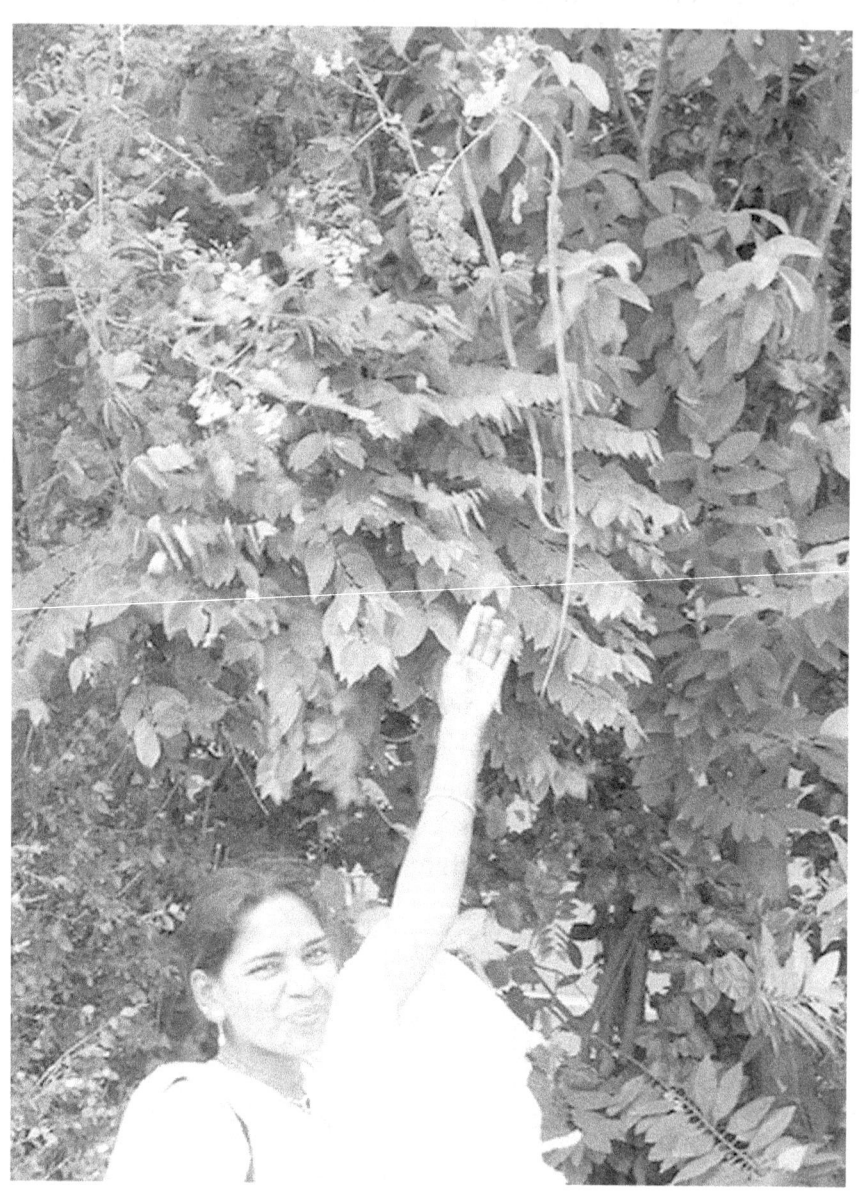

Health Benefits of Moringa

Helps in managing weight

Protects liver against damage and infection

Helps in treating cancer such as ovarian cancer

Aids in treatment of neurodegenerative diseases

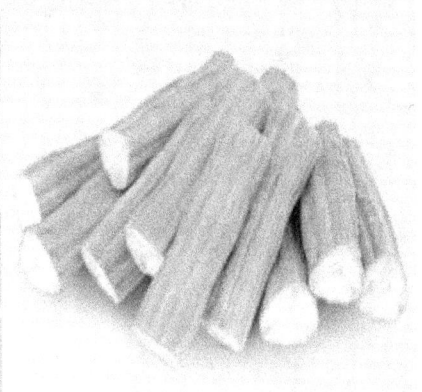

Helps to treat sickle cell disease and protects against retinal damage

Stimulates hair growth and aids in wound healing	Prevents formation of stones in kidney and bladder
Prevents wrinkles and slows premature aging of skin	Aids in treating edema, anemia, asthma and arthritis

Rich in antioxidant, antibiotic and immuno suppressive properties

Rich in anti-allergenic, antifungal and anti-fertility properties	Effective against infection caused by herpes simplex virus
Beneficial in managing diabetes and maintaining healthy heart	Effective in treating abdominal disorders such as constipation

Protects against food-borne microorganisms such as Salmonella and E. Coli

INTRODUCTION

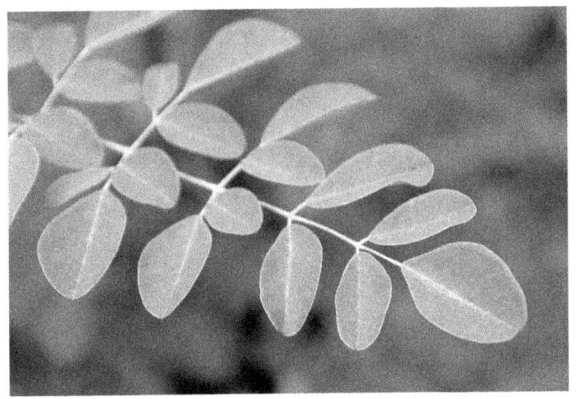

The first time I ever heard of the Moringa Tree I was doing some surfing on the internet, reading up on a variety of different kinds of nutritional information. My new journey into nutrition had just begun and I had only just discovered these strange Phytonutrient things. But they were soon to become my most consuming passion. Still, what I had learned about the Moringa Tree had made an impression. I never forgot about all the amazing things I had discovered about this "Miracle Tree of Life." It kept playing on my mind, and when my friend Robbie could not find any real science on the Moringa tree I knew that the time had come to write a book about this most amazing member of the plant kingdom!

I cannot help but to marvel at the number of different names that the Moringa Oleifera is known by in different parts of the world. We call it the Horseradish Tree, the Drumstick Tree, Mother's Best Friend, The Tree of life, as well as many more. It is loved and appreciated all over the world for its healing and curative properties. One name I am most partial to is the name by which is it most commonly known in the northern African regions. There it is called "Nebedaye," which literally means "never die" in many African languages. The Moringa plant is native to Northern India, where it was first described by native peoples around 2000 BC (that is some 4000 years ago!) as a medicinal herb. Another name for Moringa Oleifera that I really like is The Miracle Tree.

As you will see, it is a miracle indeed!

1   MEET MORINGA

The Moringa Oleifera tree, grown mainly in tropical or arid locations, has long been a source of health and vitality for the people of what we in the West call the Third

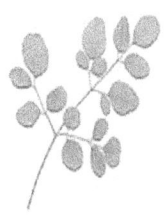

100g Moringa Dry Leaf =

10 times the Vitamin A of Carrots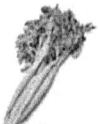

½ time the Vitamin C of Oranges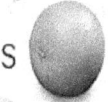

17 times the Calcium of Milk

15 times the Potassium of Bananas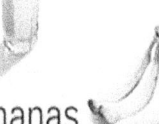

25 times the Iron of Spinach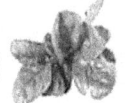

9 times the Protein of Yoghurt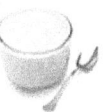

These figures reflect gram-for-gram comparisons with Moringa leaves.

World, but the usefulness of this slender tree has not been widely known here in the United States or much of the West.

The Moringa tree spread eastward from India to the lower parts of China, then to Southeast Asia, to Thailand and the over the water to the Philippines. From India It also spread westward to Egypt, then to the Horn of Africa, soon it made its way around the Mediterranean, and eventually it made the trek to the West Indies which meant it had finally arrived in the New World.

The Moringa tree is grown mainly in semiarid, tropical, and subtropical areas, corresponding in the United States to USDA hardiness zones 9 and 10. I have, however, had moderate success in zone 8 but care must be taken when winter hits! While it grows best in dry, sandy soil, it tolerates poor soil very well. In fact, the only soil that I have found that it does not really care for is good soil!

This Drumstick tree is a fast-growing, deciduous drought-resistant tree. It can grow to a height of 32–40 ft. and the trunk can reach a diameter of a foot and a half thick. The bark has a whitish-grey color and is surrounded by thick cork. Young shoots have purplish or greenish-white, hairy bark. The tree has an open crown of drooping, fragile branches and the leaves build up a feathery foliage of tripinnate leaves.

The flowers are fragrant and bisexual, surrounded by five unequal, thinly veined, yellowish-white petals. The flowers are about a 1/2" long and about 3/4" broad. They grow on slender, hairy stalks in a spreading or drooping form. Flowering usually begins within the first six months after planting. In seasonally cool regions, flowering only occurs once a year, most often between April and June. In more constant seasonal temperatures and with adequate rainfall, flowering can happen twice yearly or even all year-round.

The fruit is a hanging, three-sided brown capsule of 10 to 20 inches in size which, when opened, is found to hold dark brown, globular seeds with a diameter around half of an inch. The seeds have three whitish papery "wings" attached and are dispersed easily by both wind and water. On Moringa tree farms, the tree is habitually cut back every year to about 3 foot to 6-foot-tall and then allowed to regrow. This is so that the pods and leaves remain within arm's reach for easy harvesting.

Ancient Egyptians treasured Moringa oil, using it for their skin both as a soothing balm and as protection from the ravages of the desert weather that daily beat upon their bodies. It was well loved by men and women in all social classes in Egypt. Equally acceptable as a gift for laborer or pharaoh! How many things can you say that about?!! Later, the Greeks found many additional healthful uses for Moringa and introduced it to the Romans who carried the knowledge of Moringa oil to all parts of Europe.

On the Island of Jamaica in 1817, a petition concerning Moringa oil was presented to the Jamaican House of Assembly. It described the oil as being useful for salads and culinary purposes, as well as being equal to the best Florence oil as an illuminant – giving clear light without smoke when used in a lamp. The House declared it a national treasure!

Although not well known as yet, in The United States, the word is fast getting out. Just as the acai berry and the pomegranate became vastly popular as word of their many health benefits spread, the potent mix of antioxidants and nutrients in Moringa Oleifera is making an impact on people who are interested in increased health, vitality, and general well-being.

In addition to the high concentration of nutrients and vitamins it provides, Moringa also has been shown to increase concentration and mental focus, boost energy, increase stamina, balance emotions, and help with weight loss.

Vitamin & Mineral Content of Moringa		
All values are per 100 grams of edible portions		
	Fresh Leaves	Dried Leaves
Vitamin A	6.78 mg	18.9 mg
Niacin (B3)	0.8 mg	8.2 mg
Riboflavin (B2)	0.05 mg	20.5 mg
Thiamine (B1)	0.06 mg	2.64 mg
Vitamin C	220 mg	17.3 mg
Calcium	440 mg	2,003 mg
Carbohydrates	12.5 g	38.2 g
Protein	6.70 g	27.1 g
Calories	92 cal	205 cal
Copper	0.07 mg	0.57 mg
Fat	1.70 g	2.3 g
Fiber	0.90 g	19.2 g
Iron	0.85 mg	28.2 mg
Magnesium	42 mg	368 mg
Phosphorus	70 mg	204 mg
Potassium	259 mg	1,324 mg
Zinc	0.16 mg	3.29 mg

Unlike many plants or trees, almost all of the parts of this amazing tree are useful. The leaves, seed pods, seed pod oil, bark, stems, and roots of the Moringa tree have all been used in a medicinal or nutritional capacity for hundreds, if not thousands of years by native peoples everywhere it grows. Today, the growing and harvesting of Moringa Oleifera is a highly sustainable and environmentally friendly operation. It can be very profitable too as Moringa is second in the world only to bamboo, in growth rate.

The trees thrive in hot, sunny places, which is why most of the world's Moringa trees can be found in arid places such as Africa or Asia. Farmers and home growers typically harvest the leaves, seeds or immature seed pods, and then cut back the branches in order to stimulate rapid re-growth. Many harvesters then take the branches and compost or recycle them back into the soil in order to help improve the soil as well as to promote the heath of the land and the crop of growing trees.

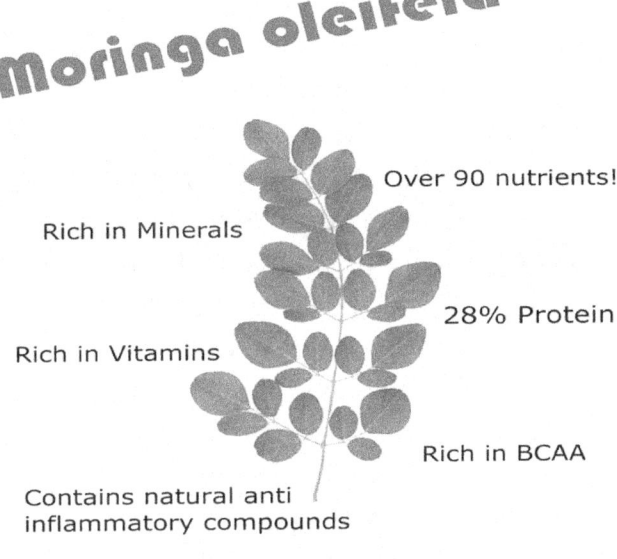

Moringa oleifera

Over 90 nutrients!

Rich in Minerals

28% Protein

Rich in Vitamins

Rich in BCAA

Contains natural anti inflammatory compounds

All essential amino acids

More antioxidants than any other plant in the world!

2 HEALTH GIVER

Often referred to as the "miracle tree" because of its uniquely diverse array of so many nutritional, medicinal, and purifying properties, the Moringa tree is a "superfood" among superfoods! It is truly a treasure with incredible potential to greatly improve health and eliminate hunger around the entire world. Because of its many valuable uses, and the fact that it grows so quickly and easily in semi-arid, tropical, and subtropical climates, the Moringa tree is quickly becoming the go-to plant for combating malnutrition, treating inflammation, promoting healthy blood flow, and preventing infection, among other things.

What is particularly unique about the Moringa tree is the fact that it is very rich in amino acids; the leaves of the Moringa tree contain 18 amino acids, eight of which are essential amino acids, making them a "complete" protein - a rarity in the plant world! Indeed, this Tree of Life's protein content rivals that of meat, making it an excellent source of protein for vegetarians and vegans.

Protein is, of course, needed to build muscle, cartilage, bones, skin and blood but it is also needed in order for the human body to be able to properly produce enzymes and hormones, important to proper human development and to a long, healthy life.

The Moringa tree's calcium and magnesium; one serving of Moringa tree leaves will provide one with approximately 125% of our recommended daily intake (RDI) of calcium and 61% of our RDI of magnesium. These two trace minerals work in synergy; while calcium is needed to build strong bones and teeth, we also need magnesium to help us better absorb the calcium. Since Moringa Oleifera contains generous quantities of both, it is especially good at guarding us from osteoporosis and other bone conditions.

The Moringa Tree nourishes the skin too; due to their trace mineral content, the dried and powdered Moringa Tree leaves are wonderful for nourishing the skin. Indeed, more and more cosmetic companies are starting to include Moringa Tree extracts in their products for this very reason. Moringa Tree creams and lotions can be applied topically on the desired areas, thus allowing the nutrients to soak into, heal, nourish, and rejuvenate, the skin.

Regularly consuming Moringa Tree leaves has also been linked to lower blood pressure, improved digestion, better mood, immune-boosting effects, and, thanks to their high fiber levels, low fat and calorie levels, weight loss.

Moringa Tree Green Superfoods Revolution

The Moringa tree pod is cooked as a vegetable in India and exported to many countries for Indian expatriates, fresh or canned. The Moringa root can be used as substitute for horseradish. Moringa foliage is eaten just like common greens, boiled, fried, and in soups or for seasoning. Dried Moringa leaf powder can be added to any kind of meal as a nutritional supplement. The Moringa tree seed can be roasted and eaten like a peanut. Moringa leaves are an inexpensive source of proteins, vitamins, and minerals for developing countries and for the rest of us too. Dried and milled, Moringa tree leaves are easily stored and used by families who can then add the powder to their daily meals. The Moringa tree powder can also be used by food businesses to enrich their products in nutrients. Moringa leaves can help decrease a developing country's dependence on imported goods, such as vitamin and mineral complexes that ward off nutritional deficiency but are too expensive to be used in a sustainably.

The Moringa Tree – A Nutritional Powerhouse

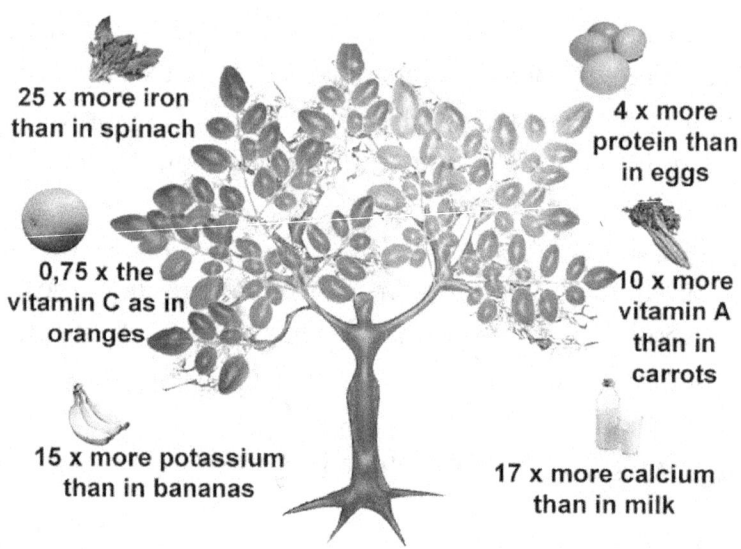

25 x more iron than in spinach

4 x more protein than in eggs

0,75 x the vitamin C as in oranges

10 x more vitamin A than in carrots

15 x more potassium than in bananas

17 x more calcium than in milk

Much of the problem with nutrition is not the quantity of food but the quality of food. This is becoming a bigger, and bigger concern to me! You need about 40 different nutrients to be healthy. Ideally, good nutrition is assured by a varied diet rich in meats, roots, grains, fruits, and vegetables. If you have a poor diet it makes you less able to resist disease, so the diseases come more frequently and they last longer. And when you get over your diarrhea or respiratory chest infection or your coughing or cold; if you are on a poor diet, you don't have the recuperative abilities of a healthy person so you don't regain the weight you have lost. In turn, you stumble from one infection to another. This has a further debilitating effect and causes depression to go along with ill health. Micronutrient deficiencies are now recognized as an important contributor to the global burden of disease.

Many people are recognizing the nutritional value of Moringa tree.

> *"Green leafy vegetables and fruits supply much needed essential micronutrients like beta-carotene [vitamin A], vitamin C, folic acid, and also calcium and potassium. Moringa Tree leaves in particular are a rich, inexpensive source of micronutrients."*

- Dr. C. Gopalan, President, Nutrition Foundation of India.

> *"Among the wide range of Green Leafy Vegetables, the Moringa tree is the richest source of Beta-Carotene [vitamin A], apart from providing other important micronutrients. Small amounts of less than 10 gm of fresh Moringa leaves would meet the day's requirement of Beta-Carotene of preschool children."*

- Dr. Kamala Krishnaswamy, Director, National Institute of Nutrition, India.

> *"As a source of nutrients and vitamins, the Moringa tree leaves rank among the best of all perennial tropical vegetables. It has been estimated that one glassful of fresh Moringa tree leaves contain the daily requirement of vitamin A for up to ten people, and adding two raw Moringa oleifera leaves to children's daily food intake, or*

mixing 2-3 teaspoons of dried Moringa tree leaf powder into other sauces living in high-risk areas." - Church World Service

"Among the leafy vegetables, one stands out as particularly good, the horseradish Moringa tree. The Moringa tree leaves are outstanding as a source of vitamin A and, when raw, vitamin C. The Moringa tree leaves are a good source of B vitamins and among the best plant sources of minerals. The calcium content is very high for a plant. Phosphorous is low, as it should be. The content of iron is very good (it is reportedly prescribed for anemia in the Philippines). Moringa leaves are an excellent source of protein and a very low source of fat and carbohydrates. Thus the Moringa tree leaves are one of the best plant foods that can be found." - Dr. Frank L. Martin, in Survival and Subsistence in the Tropics.

In his Edible Leaves of the Tropics he adds that the leaves are incomparable as a source of the sulfur-containing amino acids methionine and cystine, which are often in short supply.

According to Dr. Lowell Fuglie, the West Africa representative of the Church World Service who used the Moringa tree as a base for their most effective nutrition program:

> *"for a child aged 1-3, a 100 g serving of fresh cooked Moringa Tree leaves would provide all his daily requirements of calcium, about 75% of his iron and half his protein needs, as well as important amounts of potassium, B vitamins, copper and all the essential amino acids. As little as 20 grams of Moringa tree leaves would provide a child with all the vitamins A and C he needs."*

> *"...for pregnant and breast-feeding women, the*

Moringa leaves and pods can do much to preserve the mother's health and pass on strength and vitality to the fetus or nursing child. One 100 g portion of Moringa tree leaves could provide a woman with over a third of her daily need of calcium and give her important quantities of iron, protein, copper, sulfur and B-vitamins."
- Dr. K. MORINGA Kipling, Doctors Without Borders

"One rounded tablespoon (8 g) of Moringa Tree leaf powder will satisfy about 14% of the protein, 40% of the calcium, and 23% of the iron and nearly all the vitamin A needs for a child aged 1-3. Six rounded spoonful's of Moringa Tree leaf powder will satisfy nearly all of a woman's daily iron and calcium needs during pregnancy and breast-feeding."
- Dr. Carol Mendenhall, World Health Organization

Could Moringa leaves, leaf powder, and pods be visibly effective in treating malnutrition and promoting physical health and well-being? That was the question one European Research team posed and their results were astounding:

"Successful treatment of malnourished children has been well-documented. Interviews with men and women who have made the Moringa tree a regular part of their diets point out that they have a keen awareness of improvements in their health and energy. At one health post, the pharmacy is now selling Moringa tree leaf powder to mothers with malnourished children and the response in those children has been nothing short of miraculous!"

Another point made by the same research team was

that there is a limited awareness of nutrition and the importance of balanced diets in the under developed world. This led to the simple question:

Would people see the value of adding Moringa oleifera to their foods as a purely nutritional measure?

In the conclusion of the published research paper, in June of 2015, the team added a very important paragraph:

"It is apparent that one does not need an education in nutrition to know whether or not one is feeling healthy. People expressed every intention of continuing to include Moringa in their diets because of the sense of physical well-being it gave them. In several of the test villages, virtually every household now maintains a stock of Moringa Oleifera leaf powder. What is more in at least 3 villages the chief or elders have made consuming Moringa the law!"

Health benefits of the Moringa Tree

The Moringa tree possesses unique nutritional qualities that hold promise to millions of impoverished communities around the world that lack in many nutritional supplements such as protein, minerals, and vitamins. The Moringa leaves are an excellent source of protein that can rarely be found anywhere else, not in herbs and not in green leafy vegetables. 100g of fresh raw Moringa leaves provides 9.8g of protein or about 17.5% of RDI levels. Dry, powdered Moringa Oleifera are a much-concentrated source of many quality amino acids.

Fresh Moringa Tree pods and seeds are a good source of oleic acid, a known health-benefiting monounsaturated fat. The Moringa tree as a high-quality oilseed crop and can be grown alternatively to improve nutrition levels of populations in many drought-prone regions of Africa and

Asia.

Fresh Moringa Tree leaves and the growing tips of Moringa Trees are the richest source of vitamin A. 100g of Moringa Oleifera fresh leaves offers 7564 IU or **252% of RDI levels**. Vitamin A is one of the fat-soluble anti-oxidants found in Moringa that offers more than a few key benefits, including mucus membrane repair, maintenance of skin integrity, vision, and immunity support.

Fresh Moringa Tree pods and leaves are excellent sources of Vitamin-C too. 100g of Moringa Tree pods contains 145µg or **235%** of RDI levels of vitamin C. 10 g of greens provide 51.7µg or only 86% of RDI intake values of this important vitamin. Research studies have shown that consumption of fruits/vegetables rich in vitamin C helps the body develop immunity against infectious agents, and scavenge harmful oxygen-free radicals from the body.

The Moringa greens as well as pods contain very good amounts of many vital B-complex vitamins, including those such as folates, Vitamin-B6 (pyridoxine), thiamin (also known as Vitamin B-1), riboflavin, pantothenic acid, and niacin. Many of these vitamins function as co-enzymes in carbohydrate, protein, and fat metabolisms.

Additionally, Moringa leaves are one of the finest sources of minerals like calcium, iron, copper, manganese, zinc, selenium, and magnesium that can be found in nature. Iron alleviates anemia. Calcium, of

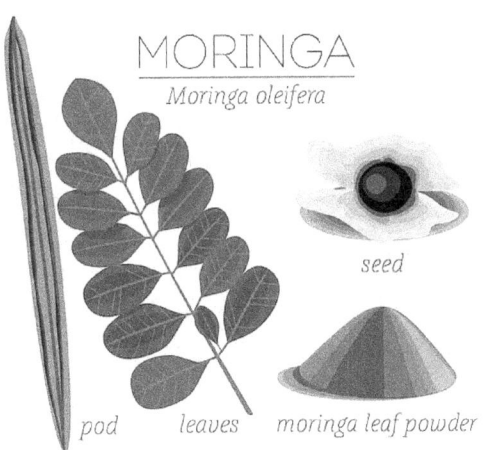

MORINGA
Moringa oleifera

seed

pod　*leaves*　*moringa leaf powder*

course, is required for bone strengthening. Zinc plays a very vital role in hair-growth, spermatogenesis, and is key to skin health.

Adoption of Moringa Tree to combat under-nutrition

Over 143 million children under the age of five in developing countries were undernourished in 2006. Food insecurity, lack of access to health care (including international food aid), and social, cultural, and economic class, all play a major role in explaining the prevalence of under-nutrition. The regions most burdened by under-nutrition, (in Africa, Asia, Latin America, and the Caribbean) all share the ability to grow and utilize the incredible, edible plant so many call the "The Tree of Life" or also commonly referred to with awe and respect, as "The Miracle Tree."

For hundreds of years, traditional healers have prescribed different parts of Moringa tree for treatment of skin diseases, respiratory illnesses, ear and dental infections, hypertension, diabetes, cancer treatment, water purification, and have promoted its use as a nutrient dense food source.

The leaves of Moringa tree have been reported to be a valuable source of both macronutrients and micronutrients and is now found growing within tropical and subtropical regions worldwide, congruent with the geographies where its nutritional benefits **are most needed.** Anecdotal evidence of benefits from the Moringa Tree has fueled a recent increase in adoption of, and attention to, its many healing benefits, specifically the high nutrient composition of the plants leaves and seeds. Once the Moringa tree leaves are harvested and cleaned, they can either be used fresh in meals or to be used at another time.

In countries that suffer from annual drought or famine before harvest season, dried Moringa Tree leaves can be made into a powder and used throughout the year. Making your own Moringa Oleifera powder fairly easy and will be discussed in Chapter 7.

There have been studies on the retention of heat sensitive vitamins, such as Vitamin A, during the drying and storage of Moringa tree leaves. For many rural agricultural societies storing grains is a common practice, and for many grains shade drying or blanching, is used prior to storage of the food source. Retention of total carotene, β-carotene, and ascorbic acid (vitamin C) was measured following storage for 2 weeks, 1, 2, and 3 months. Leaves that were blanched and sulfated compared to blanched-only leaves initially retained more total carotenes, β-carotene, and ascorbic acid but within about 3 months of storage β-carotene levels were about half of original levels in both sources, with either method of drying.

This all simply means that no matter if consumed fresh, dried, whole or ground into a powder the healing abilities of the Drumstick tree are simply astounding!

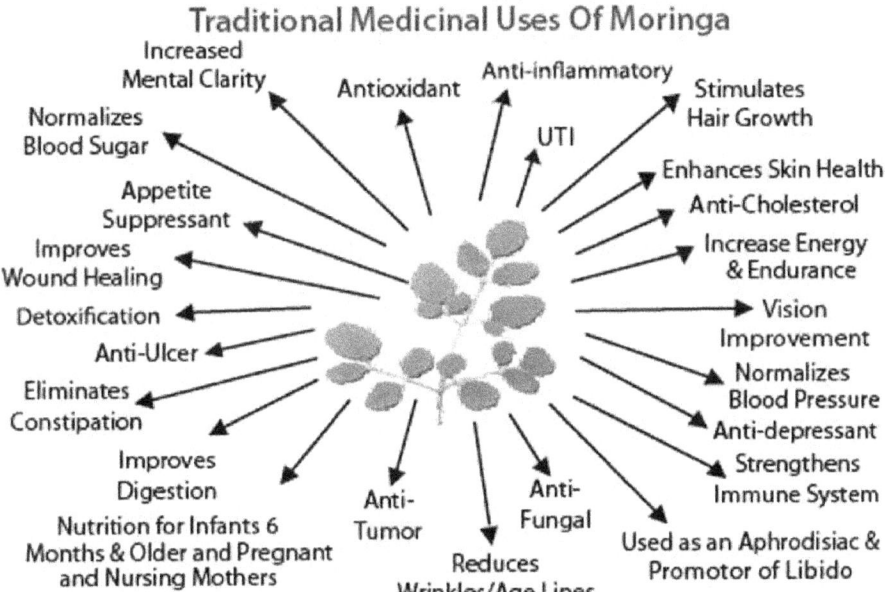

Traditional Medicinal Uses Of Moringa

Increased Mental Clarity

Antioxidant

Anti-inflammatory

Stimulates Hair Growth

Normalizes Blood Sugar

UTI

Enhances Skin Health

Anti-Cholesterol

Appetite Suppressant

Increase Energy & Endurance

Improves Wound Healing

Vision Improvement

Detoxification

Anti-Ulcer

Normalizes Blood Pressure

Eliminates Constipation

Anti-depressant

Strengthens Immune System

Improves Digestion

Anti-Tumor

Anti-Fungal

Nutrition for Infants 6 Months & Older and Pregnant and Nursing Mothers

Reduces Wrinkles/Age Lines

Used as an Aphrodisiac & Promotor of Libido

3   EASY TO GROW

As I stated earlier, the Moringa Tree is native to northern India, but today it is common to see it grown throughout the tropical and sub-tropical regions of Asia, Africa, and Latin America. Moringa trees grow easily from seeds or from cuttings. They grow very quickly even in the poorest of soils and will bloom and can be harvested as early as 8 months after planting! This is an incredible rate of growth and production and is just another reason that the Moringa Tree is favored all around the world.

To grow a Moringa Tree from a cutting:
After the trees have stopped producing fruits each year, the branches need to be cut off so that fresh, new growth may take place. These branches are excellent for using as cuttings from which to grow new trees.

1. Make a cutting at least 1" (2.5cm) in diameter and at least six feet (1.8m) long.

2. Dig a hole 3 ft. (1m) x 3 ft. (1m) and 3 ft. (1m) deep.
3. Place cutting in this hole and fill with a mixture of soil, sand and composted manure. Pack firmly around base of the cutting.
4. Form a slight dome or cone shape, sloping down away from the cutting.
5. It is desirable that water not touch the stem of the new tree.
6. Water generously, but do not drown the cutting in water.
7. In India, the custom is to put some cow dung on top of the open end of the cutting. This is an excellent way to protect the cutting from pests.

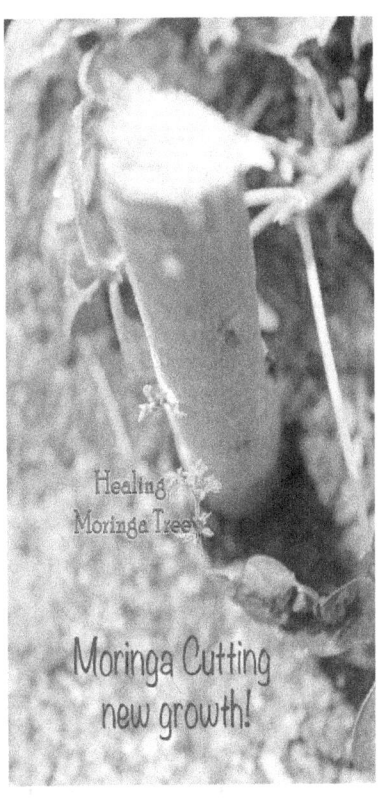

Healing
Moringa Tree

Moringa Cutting
new growth!

To grow a Moringa Tree from seed:

Moringa seeds have no dormancy periods and can be planted as soon as they are mature. It is best to plant the seeds directly where the tree is intended to grow and not transplant the seedling. The young seedlings are fragile and often cannot survive transplanting.

1. Choose an area with light and sandy soil, not heavy with clay or water-logged.
2. Dig holes 1 ft. (30 cm) square and 1 ft. deep.
3. Back-fill the holes with loose soil.

4. Compost or manure will help the tree grow better, even though Moringa trees can grow in poor soils.
5. Plant 3 to 5 seeds in each hole, 2 in. (5 cm) apart.
6. Plant the seeds no deeper than three times the width of the seed (approximately ½ in. or 1.5 cm -- the size of one's thumbnail).
7. Keep the soil moist enough so that the top soil will not dry and choke the emerging saplings, but it should not be too wet or else the seeds can drown and rot.
8. When the saplings are four to six inches tall, keep the healthiest sapling in the ground and remove the rest.
9. Termites and nematodes can kill a young sapling. Take measures to protect saplings from these two dangers.

Note: If the soil is heavy, dig a larger hole of up to 3 ft. (90 cm) in diameter and 3 ft. deep, and backfill with 1-part sand and 2 parts original soil. Added compost or manure will help.

Growing Moring in Plastic Bags or Pots:

When it is not possible to plant directly in the ground, use the following method:

1. Fill the seedling bags or pots with a light soil mixture, i.e. 3 parts soil to 1 part sand.
2. Plant two or three seeds in each bag or pot, ¼ in. (0.5 cm) deep.
3. Keep moist but not too wet. Germination will occur within two weeks.
4. Remove extra seedlings, leaving one in each bag or pot.
5. Seedlings can be transplanted after four to six months when they are 2-3 ft (60-90 cm) high.

Transplanting:

The ground where the trees are to be planted should be light and sandy, not heavy with clay or water-logged.

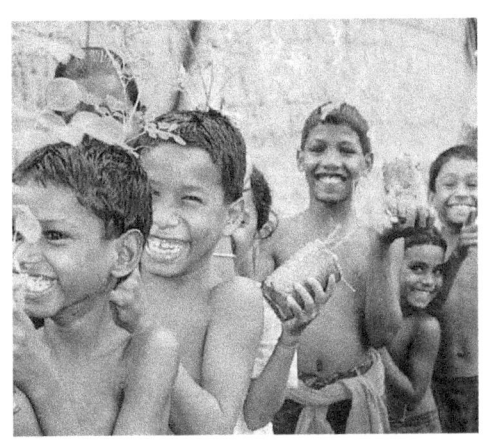

1. Dig a hole 1 ft. (30 cm) square and 1 ft. deep. Backfill with loose soil. Adding compost or manure will help the trees grow better.
2. Water the planting holes one day before transplanting the seedlings.
3. Plant seedlings in the late afternoon to avoid the hot sun the first day.
4. Make a hole in the pit to accept all soil in the bag or pot.
5. Carefully cut open the sack and place the seedling in the planting hole. Be careful to keep the soil

around the seedling's roots intact.
6. Pack soil around the seedling base.
7. Water only lightly for the first few days.
8. If the seedlings fall over, tie them to a stick for support.
9. Protect young saplings from termites and nematodes.

PLANTING THE TREE

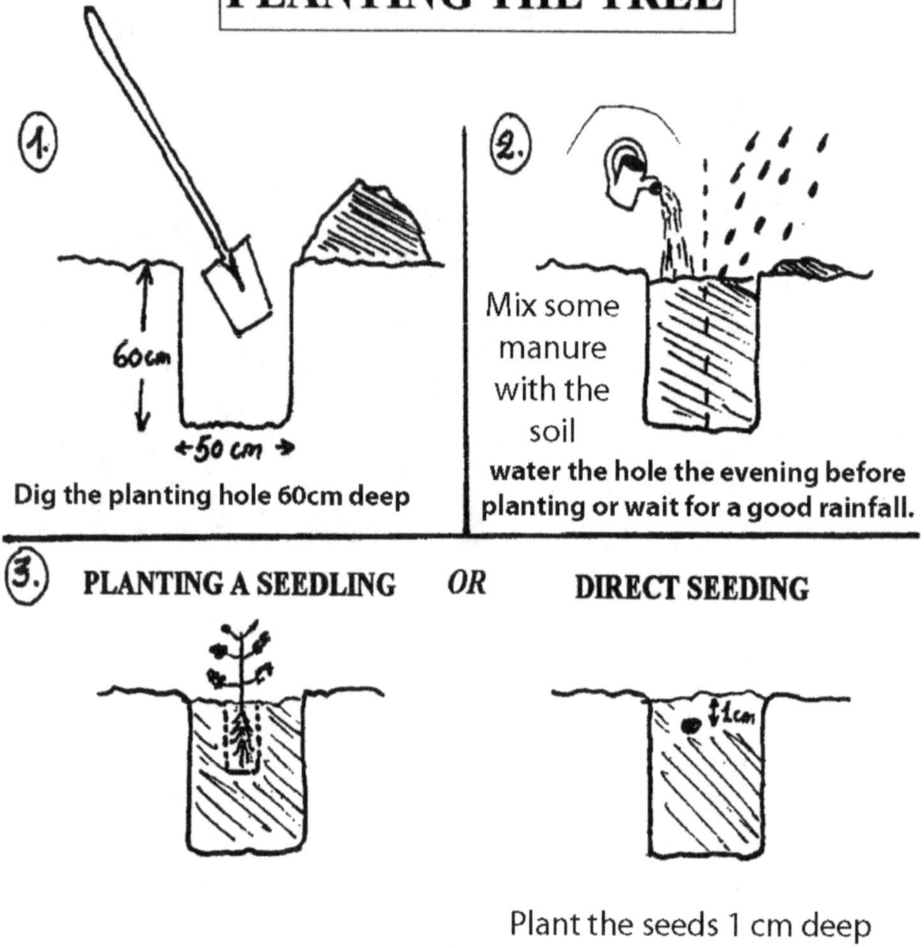

①.

60cm

←50 cm →

Dig the planting hole 60cm deep

②.

Mix some manure with the soil

water the hole the evening before planting or wait for a good rainfall.

③.   PLANTING A SEEDLING   *OR*   DIRECT SEEDING

↕1cm

Plant the seeds 1 cm deep

Why not Grow a Moringa Pharmacy?

Moringa is easy to grow so I suggest that we all **get a little Moringa in our diets by planting and using our very own multivitamin in our yard! – AND IT IS FUN TOO!!!**

What could be easier than walking into your yard, and gathering healthy leaves from your own grown Moringa plants to put on the table? The Moringa plant is fun because is so fast-growing that you can almost see a difference every day! Learn how to grow your own multivitamin and have a Moringa pharmacy at your doorstep. Simply plant seeds or cuttings in a sunny spot. (that is nearly all you have to do!!!)

So let's review growing a Moringa Pharmacy of your very own, both for beginners and those who are more expert gardeners:

Moringa Plant, Grow, Cultivation - Easy Instructions

1. Find a sunny place
2. Make square holes in the ground 30 to 60 cm deep
3. Fill the hole with loose soil
4. Plant the seed 1 cm deep
5. Give the ground some water but not too much, otherwise the seed may rotten.
6. Within 1-2 weeks the Miracle springs out the ground!

Moringa Planting, Growing, & Cultivation for the 'Expert'

Moringa Oleifera is believed to be native to sub-Himalayan tracts of northern India but is now found worldwide in the tropics and sub-tropics. It grows best in direct sunlight under 1500 feet in altitude. It tolerates a wide range of soil conditions, but prefers a neutral to slightly acidic pH (6.3-7.0). It wants well-drained sandy or loamy soil but can grow in just about any soil. Obviously it needs water but its but it grows with a varied amount of rainfall - minimum annual rainfall requirements are estimated at 10 inches but can handle as much as 118 inches – a very wide range! But it should be noted that in waterlogged soil the roots have a tendency to rot. (In areas with heavy rainfall, trees are usually planted on small hills to encourage water run-off). The presence of a long taproot makes it resistant to periods of drought. The Moringa Trees can be easily grown from seed or from cuttings. Its Temperature requirements range from 75° – 95° Fahrenheit (25°-35° Celsius) but the tree will tolerate up to 120° (48° Celsius) in the shade and it can survive a **mild** frost.

Moringa seeds have no dormancy period, so they can be planted as soon as they are mature and they will retain the ability to germinate for up to one year or so. Older seeds will only have spotty germination. Moringa Trees will flower and fruit annually and in some regions twice annually. During its first year, a Moringa Tree will grow up to 15 feet (5 meters) in height and produce flowers and fruit. Left alone, the tree can eventually reach 30 – 40 feet high (12 meters) in height with a trunk of about 15 inches or 30cm wide; however, the tree can be annually cut back to one meter from the ground. The tree will quickly recover and produce leaves and pods within easy reach. Within three years a tree will yield 400-600 pods annually and a mature tree can produce up to

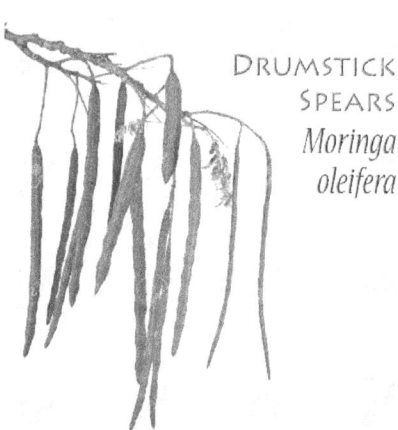

DRUMSTICK
SPEARS
Moringa
oleifera

1,600 pods. Coppicing to the ground is also possible, and will produce a Moringa bush as no main new growth is selected, and the others eliminated.

Moringa Plant, Grow, Cultivation - IN THE NURSERY

Use poly bags or pots with dimensions of about 18cm or 8" in height and 12cm or 4-5" in diameter. The soil mixture for the plantings should be light, i.e. 3 parts soil to 1 part sand. Plant two or three seeds in each sack, ½ to 1 inch deep. Keep the seeds moist **but not too wet**.

Germination will occur within 5 to 12 days, depending on the age of the seed and pre-treatment method used. Remove extra seedlings, leaving one in each sack. Seedlings can be out-planted when they are 60-90cm or 12-36 inches high. When out-planting, cut a hole in the bottom of the sack big enough to allow the roots to emerge. Be sure to retain the soil around the roots of the seedling. To encourage rapid germination, one of three pre-seeding treatments can be employed:

1. Soak the seeds in water overnight before planting.
2. Crack the shells before planting.
3. Remove shells and plant kernels only.

Moringa Plant, Grow, Cultivation - IN THE FIELD

If planting a large plot, it is recommended to first plough the land. Prior to planting a seed or seedling, dig a planting pit about 24 inches or 50cm in depth and the same in width. This planting hole serves to loosen the soil and helps to retain moisten in the root zone, enabling the seedlings' roots to develop rapidly. Compost or manure at the rate of 20% of the pit, then mix with the fresh topsoil around the hole and use to fill up the pit. Avoid using the soil taken out of the hole for this purpose: **use fresh soil that contains beneficial microbes that can promote more effective root growth**.

The day before planting, water the filled pits or wait until a good rain before out-planting seedlings. Fill in the hole before transplanting the seedling. In areas of heavy rainfall, the soil can be shaped in the form of a mound to encourage drainage. **Do not water heavily** for the first few days. If the seedlings fall over, tie them to stick about 2 foot or 40cm high for support.

Moringa Plant, Grow, Cultivation - DIRECT SEEDING
If water is available for irrigation (i.e., in a backyard garden), Moringa Trees can be seeded directly and grown anytime during the year. Prepare a planting pit first, water, and then fill in the pit with topsoil mixed with compost or manure before planting seeds. In a large field, trees can be seeded directly at the beginning of the wet season.

Moringa Plant, Grow, Cultivation - GROWING MORINGA FROM CUTTINGS
Use hard wood, not green wood, for cuttings. Cuttings should be about 20 inches or more in length (45cm to 1.5m long). Cuttings can be planted directly or planted in sacks in the nursery. When planting directly, plant the cuttings in light, sandy soil. Plant one-third of the length in the ground (i.e., if the cutting is 1.5m long, plant it 50cm deep). Do not over water; if the soil is too heavy or wet, the roots may rot. When the cuttings are planted in the nursery, the root system is slow to develop. Add phosphorus to the soil if possible to encourage root development. Cuttings

planted in a nursery can be out-planted after 2 or 3 months.

Moringa Plant, Grow, Cultivation - SPACING

For intensive Moringa production, plant the tree every 9 feet or 3 meters in rows 9 feet or 3 meters apart. To ensure sufficient sunlight and airflow, it is also recommended that one plant the trees in an east-west direction. When the trees are part of an alley-cropping system, there should be 30 feet or 10 meters between the rows. The area between trees should be kept free of weeds and lightly mulched.

Trees are often spaced in a line one meter or less apart in order to create living fence posts, this is fine just keep in mind that the trees will not grow as tall when planted in this fashion. Trees are also planted to provide support for climbing crops such as pole beans, although only mature trees should be used for this purpose since the vine growth can choke off the young tree.

Here is a Great Idea for you:

Moringa Trees can be planted in gardens where they can benefit the other garden vegetables! How? Well, the tree's root system is very deep and so It does not compete with most other garden crops for surface nutrients and the dapple shade it will provide can be used to the benefit of those veggies that are less tolerant of direct, hot sunlight!

From the second year onwards, Moringa trees can be inter-cropped with corn, sunflower and other field crops. Sunflower is particularly recommended for helping to control weed growth. However, Moringa Trees are reported to be highly competitive with many eggplant and some sweet corn, and can reduce their yields by up to 50%.

Moringa Plant, Grow, Cultivation - PINCHING THE TERMINAL TIPS

When the seedlings reach a height of 2 ½ feet (60cm) in the main field, pinch (trim) the terminal growing tip 5 or 6 inches (10cm) from the top. This can be done using fingers since the terminal growth is still very green and tender, devoid of bark fiber and quite brittle, and therefore easily broken. A shears or knife blade can also be used. Secondary branches will begin appearing on the main stem below the cut about a week later. When they reach a length of about 10 to 12 inches (20cm), cut these back by half. Use a sharp blade and make a slanting cut. Tertiary branches will appear, and these are also to be pinched in the same manner. This pinching, done four times before the flowers appear (when the tree is about three months old), will encourage the tree to become bushy and produce many pods within easy reach. Pinching helps the tree develop a strong production frame for maximizing the yield. If the pinching is not done, the tree has a tendency to shoot up vertically and grow tall, like a mast, with sparse flowers and few fruits found only at the very top. Those are very difficult to harvest!

For annual Moringa types, directly following the end of the harvest, cut the tree's main trunk to about 3 to 4 foot or 90cm from ground level. About two weeks later 15 to 20 sprouts will appear below the cut. Allow only 4-5 robust branches to grow and nib the remaining sprouts while they are young, before they grow long and harden. Continue the same pinching process as done with new seedlings so as to make the tree bushy.

Moringa Plant, Grow, Cultivation - WATERING

Moringa trees do not need much watering, which make them ideally suited for the climate of places such as Southern California. In very dry conditions, water regularly for the first two months and afterwards only when the tree is obviously suffering. Moringa trees will flower and produce pods whenever there is sufficient rainfall or other water available. If rainfall is continuous throughout the year,

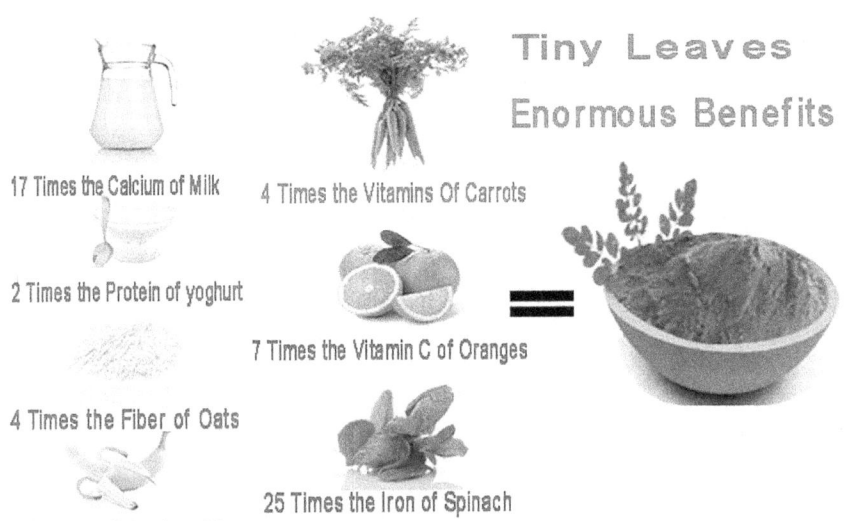

Tiny Leaves
Enormous Benefits

17 Times the Calcium of Milk

4 Times the Vitamins Of Carrots

2 Times the Protein of yoghurt

7 Times the Vitamin C of Oranges

4 Times the Fiber of Oats

25 Times the Iron of Spinach

15 Times the Potassium of Bananas

Moringa trees will have a nearly continuous yield. In arid conditions, flowering can be induced through irrigation.

Moringa Plant, Grow, Cultivation - FERTILIZING

Moringa trees will generally grow well without adding very much additional fertilizer. Manure or compost can be mixed with the soil used to fill the planting pits. Phosphorus can be added to encourage root development and nitrogen will encourage leaf canopy growth. In some parts of India, 15cm-deep ring trenches are dug about 10cm from the trees during the rainy season and filled with green leaves, manure and ash. These trenches are then covered with soil.

This approach is said to promote higher pod yields. Research done in India has also showed that applications of 7.5kg farmyard manure and 0.37kg ammonium sulfate per tree can increase pod yields threefold. Biodynamic composts yield the best results, with yield increases of to 50% compared to ordinary composts.

Moringa is resistant to most pests. In very water-logged conditions, Diplodia root rot can occur. In very wet conditions, seedlings can be planted in mounds so that excess water is drained off. Cattle, sheep, pigs and goats will eat Moringa seedlings, pods and leaves. Protect Moringa seedlings from livestock by installing a fence or by planting a living fence around the plantation. For mature trees, the lower branches can be cut off so that goats or deer will not be able to reach the leaves and pods.

In some parts of the world termites can be a problem, among approaches recommended to protect seedlings from termite attack:

1. Apply mulches of castor oil plant leaves, mahogany chips, tephrosia leaves or Persian lilac leaves around the base of the plants.
2. Heap ashes around the base of seedlings.
3. Dry and crush stems and leaves of lion's ear or Mexican poppy and spread the dust around the base of plants.

In India, various caterpillars are reported to cause defoliation unless controlled by spraying. Elsewhere in the world, where Moringa is an introduced tree, local pests are less numerous and fewer problems are reported.

Moringa Plant, Grow, Cultivation - HARVESTING

When harvesting pods for human consumption, harvest when the pods are still young (about a ½ inch or 1cm in diameter) and snap easily. Older pods develop a tough exterior, but the white seeds and flesh remain edible until the ripening process begins.

When producing seed for planting or for oil extraction, allow the pods to dry and turn brown on the tree. In some cases, it may be necessary to prop up a branch that holds many pods to prevent it breaking off. Harvest the pods before they split open and seeds fall to the ground. Seeds can be stored in well-ventilated sacks in dry, shady places for over a year.

For making leaf based sauces, harvest seedlings, growing tips, or young leaves. Older leaves must be stripped from the tough and wiry stems. These older leaves are more suited to making dried leaf powder since the stems are removed in the pounding and sifting process.

Moringa Compared to 100gm. Edible Portion of Common Foods from *Nutritive Value of Indian Foods* by C.Gopalan, et al.		
Nutrient	Moringa	Other Foods
Vitamin A	6780 mcg	Carrots: 1890 mcg
Vitamin C	220 mg	Oranges: 30 mg
Calcium	440 mg	Cow's milk: 120 mg
Potassium	259 mg	Bananas: 88 mg
Protein	6.7 gm	Cow's milk: 3.2 gm

4   BOTANICAL DESCRIPTION

Moringa is a slender softwood tree that branches freely and can be extremely fast growing. Although it can reach heights in excess of 10m (33ft), it is generally considered to be a small to medium size tree. Tripinnate compound leaves are feathery with green to dark green elliptical leaflets of about 2cm (0.5 – 1 inch) in length. The tree is often mistaken for a legume because of its leaves and conspicuous, lightly fragmented flowers that are generally white to cream colored, although they can be tinged with pink in some varieties. The fruit is a tri-lobed capsule and is frequently referred to as a 'pod'. Immature pods are green and in some varieties have some reddish color.

The fast growing, drought-tolerant Moringa Oleifera can tolerate seriously poor soil, a wide rainfall range and a soil ph from 5.0 – 9.0. All of this means that it can be grown just about anywhere in just about any soil!

When fully mature, dried seeds are round or triangular shaped and the kernel is surrounded by a lightly wooded shell with three papery wings. Moringa Oleifera seeds contain between 33% and 41% vegetable oil. Research has determined that the composition of Moringa Oleifera, what with its fatty acid profile, is high in oleic acid. The seeds contain around 70% – 85% oleic oil, which has been identified as being a very good source of biofuel as well as having great medicinal value.

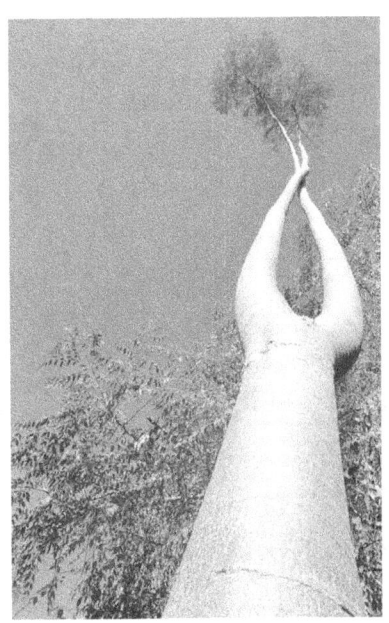

Parts of the tree

- **Stem:** The Stem is normally straight but has been known to occasionally form twisted or curved. The tree grows with a short, straight stem that reaches a height of 5-6 feet before it begins branching but can reach up to 9 feet.

- **Branch**: The extended branches grow in a disorganized, seemingly random manner that never the less leads to an umbrella shaped canopy.
- **Leaves**: Tripinnate compound leaves are feathery with green to dark green elliptical leaflets about ½ an inch to one-inch long. The tree is often mistaken for a legume because of its leaves. The alternate twice or thrice pinnate leaves grow mostly at the branch tips. They are 10–30 inches long and grayish-green when young.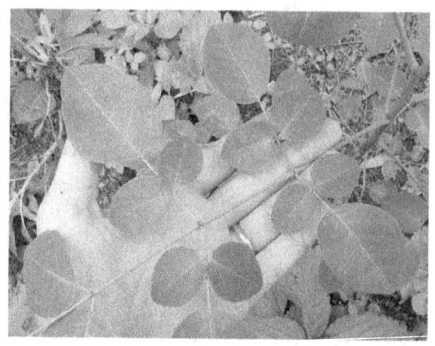
- **Flowers**: The conspicuous, lightly fragrant flowers are borne on inflorescences about 6-12 inches long, and are generally white to cream colored, an inch or so in diameter, borne in sprays, with 5 at the top of the flower, 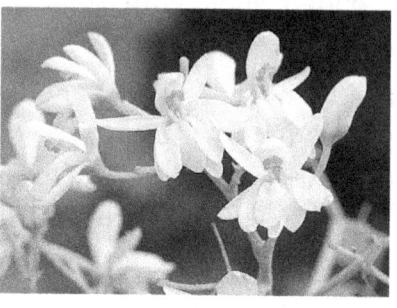 although they can be tinged with pink in some varieties. The flowers, which are pleasantly fragrant and 1-2 inches wide are produced profusely in auxiliary, dropping panicles 6-12 inches long. They are white or cream colored and yellow dotted at the base. The flowers are very attractive and provide a pleasant fragrance.

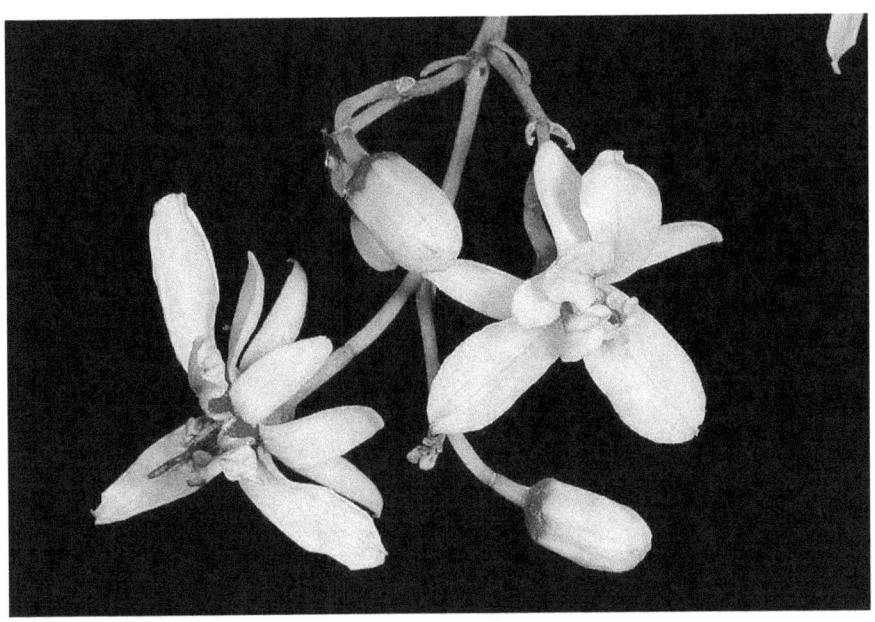

- **Fruits**: The fruits are tri-lobed capsules, and are frequently referred to as pods. Immature pods are green and in some varieties have some reddish color. The pods are pendulous, brown, triangular, splitting lengthwise into 3 parts when dry, containing about 20 or so seeds embedded in the pith.

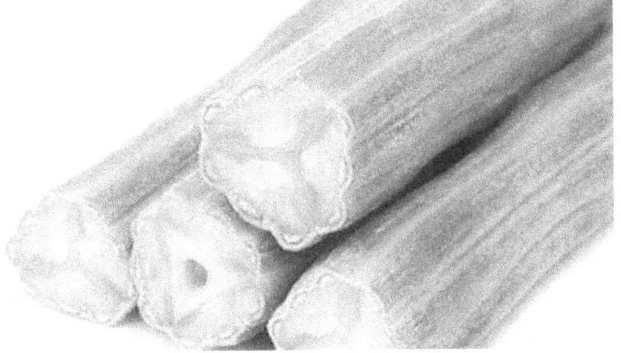

- **Seeds**: The seed are round with a brownish semi-permeable seed hull; each has 3 papery wings connected. The seed hulls are generally brown to black, but can be white if kernels are of low viability. Viable seeds germinate within a week.

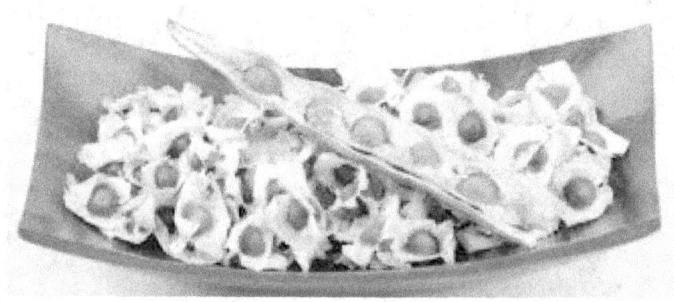

ENVIRONMENTAL PREFERENCES AND TOLERANCE

Moringa oleifera can grow at a remarkable rate when young with 9 to 12 feet of growth in the first year not being unusual when growing in favorable conditions. In cultivation, trees raised from seed start flowering after 2 years of growth while trees grown from large cuttings can begin to produce fruit some six to twelve months after planting.

Mature trees can eventually reach a height of 18 – 40 feet high when growing in good conditions in the wild. However, plants growing in marginal, conditions grow much slower and can have a stunted and shrubby habit sometimes only reaching 10 - 12 feet in height. Trees grown on tree farms are most often kept pruned to just 6 – 10 feet high to allow for easier harvesting of leaves and pods.

The Moringa tree may drop its leaves during the dry season and relies on the fact that it has an enlarged underground rootstock (tap root) to find water. These two characteristics make it very drought tolerant, it performs extremely well in even severe drought conditions and is often among the first plants to rebound when conditions improve. In the northern hemisphere, the Miracle tree loses its leaves from December to January, though during droughts it may also lose its leaves at other times of the year. New growth usually begins to appear in February or March and flowering often precedes or coincides with the appearance of the new leaves.

The bisexual flowers of Moringa Oleifera are highly cross-pollinated and pollination is mainly facilitated by animals, that is to say that the flowers are zoophilous (man, I love that crazy word!!) but again, it can also self-pollinate.

For example, bees, butterflies and birds have been observed to be very active and reliable pollinators in most parts of the world. The Drumstick tree does not seem to require any specific pollinators as it readily produces viable seed in all parts of the world where it had been introduced (including most recently in the United States and Australia).

During one study on the mating system of the Tree of Life, it was found that 74% of the seed were produced as a result of cross-pollination and the remaining 26% of seed were produced by self-fertilization. While these rates may be influenced by a number of environmental factors, this study confirms that Moringa Oleifera has a mixed mating system and is capable of reproducing from a single individual. Which means that even if you only have a single tree planted you will still get fruit and can reap

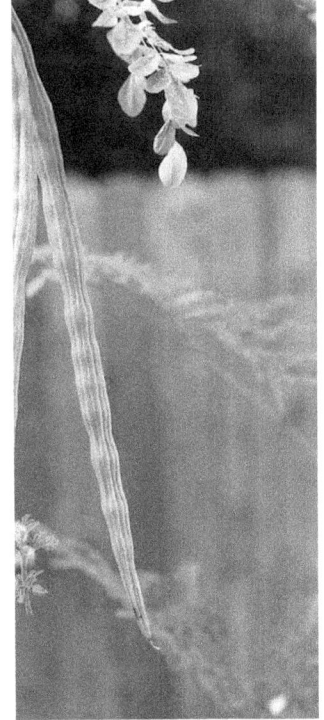

all of the health benefits this wonder of nature has to offer.

A single tree can produce 300 to 400 fruit per year within 3 years of planting while a mature tree can produce up to 1000 fruit, or more, per year. As each Fruit contains approximately 20 seeds, a mature tree can therefore produce 20,000 or more seeds per year.

5 NUTRITIONAL PROPERTIES OF MORINGA OLEIFERA

In several developing tropical countries, Moringa trees have been used to combat malnutrition, especially among infants and nursing mothers.

In fact, three non-governmental organizations in particular; *Trees for Life, Church World Service,* and *The Educational Concerns for Hunger Organization* all advocate moringa as a 'natural nutrition for the tropics'.

The Leaves of this amazing tree can be eaten fresh, cooked or stored as a dried powder for many months without refrigeration or loss of nutritional value. This alone sets Moringa Oleifera apart from many other plants. Moringa is especially, promising as a food source in the tropics because the tree is in full leaf at the end of the dry season while other foods are typically still very scare. Research analyses of the leaf's composition has revealed them to have significant quantities of the Vitamins A, B and C, as well as high counts of calcium, iron and protein.

According to *Optima of Africa ltd*, a group that has been working with the Miracle Tree in Tanzania for over a dozen years, just 25 grams daily of moringa leaf powder will provide a child the following recommended daily allowances:

- protein   42%
- calcium   125%
- magnesium 61%
- potassium 41%
- iron   71%
- vitamin A 272%
- vitamin C 22%

These numbers are particularly astounding, considering this nutrition is available when other food sources are usually very scarce.

Some further research analyses of the composition of

Supplement Facts
Serving Size: 1 scoop (8 grams)

	Amount Per Serving	%DV
Calories	21 g	†
Protein	2.3 g	5%
Fat	0.5 g	1%
Sugar	0.06 g	#
Dietary Fiber	4.0 g	16%
Vitamin A	1480 IU	30%
Vitamin B1	0.04 mg	3%
Vitamin B2	0.1 mg	6%
Vitamin B6	0.13 mg	7%
Vitamin B12	0.06 µg	1%
Vitamin E	5.15 mg	31%
Sodium	13 mg	1%
Potassium	0.15 g	4%
Calcium	0.13 g	13%
Magnesium	43 mg	11%
Iron	2.7 mg	1%
Phosphorus	26 mg	3%

† Percent Daily Value not established.

the Drumstick Tree seeds has shown high levels of lipids and proteins. They have described high levels of total proteins, which are even higher than in important legume seeds when it comes to human nutrition. The dry legume seeds usually contain between 18% to 25% protein, nearly double the contents of cereal grains, Moringa contains up to 42% protein. The seed lipid content of Moringa seeds is even greater than that of most soybean varieties; which are used to produce over 75% of all vegetable oils in the United States.

The major saturated fatty acids present in the seeds are palmitic stearic, arachidic and benic acids. Oleic acid is the major unsaturated fatty acid whose high concentration is desirable in terms of nutrition and stability during cooking and frying. Moreover, as a natural source of benic acid, the Moringa Oleifera seed oil has been used as a solidifying agent in margarines and other food stuffs containing solid and semi solid fat, therefore eliminating hydrogenation processes. Pods contain irrelevant amounts of tannins but saponins and alkaloids are present in amounts biologically important in the leaves and stems, respectively, although in levels considered nontoxic to ruminants.

A large number of reports on the nutritional qualities of Moringa now exist in both scientific and popular literature. Any readers who are familiar with Moringa will recognize the oft produced characterization made many years ago by the *Trees for Life* organization, that:

> *"ounce for ounce, moringa leaves contains more vitamin A than carrots, more calcium than milk, more iron than spinach, more vitamin C than an orange and more potassium than bananas, and that the protein quality of moringa leaves rivals that of milk and eggs."*

The reader will also recognize the oral histories recorded by Lowell Fuglie, in Senegal and throughout west Africa, who reports on (and has extensively documented on video) countless instances of lifesaving nutritional rescues that are attributed almost exclusively to Moringa Oleifera consumption. In fact, the nutritional properties of Moringa are now so well known that there seems to be little doubt of substantial health benefits to be realized through the consumption of Moringa leaf, leaf powder, and other parts of the Moringa Tree, especially in situations where starvation is imminent. Nevertheless, the outcome of well controlled and well documented clinical studies are still coming in and are still clearly of great value.

MORINGA OLEIFERA

Why should I take Moringa Oleifera Products?

- Research has proved that various parts of the **Moringa tree** can be used to prevent and cure a minimum of 300 diseases
- **Moringa** contains more than 90 nutrients and 46 types of antioxidants
- The problem with nutrition is not the quantity of food, but the quality of food we eat, with people needing about 40 different nutrients to be healthy. Lack of quality foods is malnutrition. **Moringa Leaves** has 90+ verifiable nutrients and not only contains all these elements, but also has significant portions of Vitamins B, B1, B2, B3, D, and E, antioxidants, other minerals, fibre and is one of the highest, naturally occurring sources of chlorophyll
- The proteins in **Moringa Leaves** gives 18 of the 20 known amino acids, including all eight amino acids classified as essential. These essential amino acids cannot be synthesized by the body and must come from a person's diet, usually from red meat or dairy products. These foods are not available in many parts of the world and are lacking in the diets of vegetarians, elderly people, and children
- Vitamins and other nutrients are best absorbed and used by the body when they are derived from natural sources like **Moringa Leaves** and are present in naturally occurring complex compounds

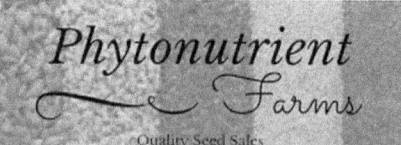

Phytonutrient Farms
Quality Seed Sales

The Moringa tree contains many nutrients such as essential vitamins, essential minerals, necessary amino acids, beta-carotene, antioxidants and inflammatory nutrients, phytonutrients and, incredibly, it also contains both omega-3 and omega-6 fatty acids.

<u>This is huge! This is incredible!</u>
<u>This is amazingly rare!</u>

The leaves are highly nutritive, being a significant source of beta-carotene, Vitamin C, protein, iron, and potassium. The leaves can be cooked and used like spinach, or used washed and raw in a salad. In addition to being used fresh as a substitute for greens, its leaves are commonly dried and crushed into powder and used in soups, stews, and sauces. The tree is a good source of calcium and phosphorus, Moringa leaves and pods are helpful in increasing breast milk yield for nursing mothers during the breast feeding months of her new child's life. Incredibly, just one tablespoon of leaf powder can provide 14% of the protein, 40% of the calcium, 23% of the iron and most of the Vitamin A needs of a child aged one to three years. Six table spoons of leaf powder will provide nearly all of the woman's daily iron and calcium needs during pregnancy and breastfeeding!

All her needs and all naturally! How cool is that?!

The Moringa seeds yield 38%-40% edible oil. The refined oil is clear, odorless and resists rancidity at least as well as any other botanical oil. The seedcake remaining after oil extraction may be used as fertilizer or as a flocculent that forms the particles into a solid so that it can be used to purify water. Yes, you read that correctly, basically, the waste product of making the precious Moringa oil from the seeds of the Moringa tree can then be used to purify water for both humans and livestock consumption! **Are you beginning to see why this tree has been called a Miracle?!!**

It is well known and well documented that nutrients and phytonutrients are very important for human health and vitality. Because Moringa Oleifera contains so many essential nutrients and phytonutrients in virtually all the different parts of the tree, Moringa is considered a true treasure and a blessing in much of the world. Towns and villages all over the globe are using different parts of the tree for a variety of nutritional, medicinal and purification purposes. Even the root of the tree is used, though sparingly as it is advisable not to consume the roots in great quantity since researchers have determined that the root can be toxic and contains chemicals that can paralyze nerves. Moringa Oleifera is sometimes referred to as the 'tree of life' because of its potential to help with malnutrition around the world. Given its nutritional value, it can be utilized in fortifying sauces, juices, spices, milk, bread and most importantly for

Supplement Facts

Serving Size: ½ teaspoon (1g)
Servings Per Container: about 225

Amount Per Serving

Calories 3	Calories from Fat 0	
		% Daily Value*
Total Fat 0g		0%
Saturated Fat 0g		0%
Trans Fat 0g		
Cholesterol 0mg		0%
Sodium 0mg		0%
Potassium 18mg		<1%
Total Carbohydrate 1g		0%
Dietary Fiber <1g		0%
Sugars 0g		
Protein <1g		
Vitamin A 5%	•	Vitamin C 15%
Calcium 3%	•	Iron 5%
Thiamin 110%	•	Riboflavin 130%
Vitamin B12 106%		

Organic Moringa Leaf (Moringa oleifera) †

*Percent Daily Values are based on a 2,000 calorie diet.
†Daily value not established.

GLUTEN FREE · GMO FREE · KOSHER

Contains No: sugar, salt, starch, yeast, wheat, corn, soy, milk, egg, shellfish or preservatives. Vegetarian/Vegan Product.

Certified Organic by Control Union

AMINO ACID PROFILE

Alanine	7.66 mg
Arginine	32.0 mg
Aspartic Acid	2.23 mg
Cystine	4.06 mg
Glutamic acid	1.79 mg
Glycine	52.1 mg
Histidine	0.10 mg
Isoleucine	1.56 mg
Leucine	0.18 mg
Lysine	3.46 mg
Methionine	9.16 mg
Phenylalanine	0.18 mg
Proline	5.78 mg
Serine	0.01 mg
Threonine	38.5 mg
Tryptophan	0.21 mg
Tyrosine	45.1 mg
Valine	94.9 mg
Total Amino Acids	299.21 mg

Distributed in the USA by: Organic India USA
5311 Western Ave., Suite 110,
Boulder, CO 80301
888-550-8332
PRODUCT OF INDIA

ORGANIC
INDIA™

MAKERS of the
ORIGINAL TULSI TEAS™

much of the planet, instant noodles. Many commercial products like Zija brand soft drinks, tea and nutraceuticals are now including Moringa in their recipes and are available all over the globe.

A comparative study of Moringa fresh leaves gram for gram with other foodstuffs puts Moringa on the top of the list; it contains seven times the Vitamin C of oranges, four times the Vitamin A of carrots, four times the calcium of milk, three times the potassium of bananas and two times the protein of yogurt. But the micro nutrient content is even greater in the dried leaves, ten times the Vitamin A of carrots, 17 times the calcium of milk, 15 times the potassium of bananas, 25 times the iron of spinach, and nine times the protein of yoghurt, however the Vitamin C drops to half that of oranges in the dried leaves. This tree is truly a "miracle" tree offering hope, nutritionally, medicinally and economically to devastatingly poor 3rd world countries and it has just begun being used as a dietary supplement by growing numbers of in the West.

Recently, a high degree of renewed interest was placed on the nutritional properties of Moringa in most countries where it was not native. This could be due to the fact that it increases herd animal productivity as it has nutritional, therapeutic and prophylactic properties. Studies from many western countries indicate that the leaves have immense nutritional value such as vitamins, minerals and amino acids that can benefit livestock. As such, the leaves have been used to combat malnutrition, especially among infants in large herds. Amino acids, fatty acids, minerals and vitamins are as essential in animal feed as they are to human beings.

These nutrients are used for osmotic adjustment, activate enzymes, hormones and other organic molecules that enhance growth, function and enhance the animals' quality of life.

If you have a science background you may find the tables on the following pages interesting, I did!

Chemical composition of dried leaves of Moringa Oleifera

Nutritive value	Dry leaf	Standard error
Moisture (%)	9.533	0.194
Crude protein (%)	30.29	1.480
Fat (%)	6.50	1.042
Ash (%)	7.64	0.433
Neutral detergent fibre(%)	11.40	0.425
Acid detergent fibre(%)	8.49	0.348
Acid detergent lignin(%)	1.8	2.204
Acid detergent cellulose(%)	4.01	0.101
Condensed tannins(mg/g)	3.12	0.104
Total polyphenols(%)	2.02	0.390

Source: (Busani, MORINGA, Patrick, J. MORINGA, Arnold, H. and Voster, MORINGA (2011)

Moringa Leaves - Nutritional Value Per Gram As compared to everyday food!

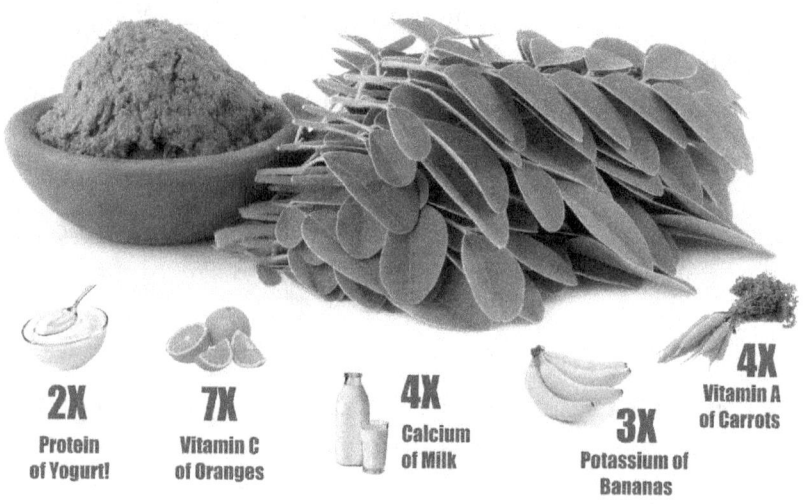

2X Protein of Yogurt!

7X Vitamin C of Oranges

4X Calcium of Milk

3X Potassium of Bananas

4X Vitamin A of Carrots

Amino acids composition of dried Moringa leaves

Amino acid	Quantity (mean +/- %)	Standard error
Argenine	1.78	0.010
Serine	1.087	0.035
Aspartic acid	1.43	0.045
Glutamic acid	2.53	0.062
Glycine	1.533	0.060
Threonine	1.357	0.124
Alanine	3.033	0.006
Tyrosine	2.650	0.015
Proline	1.203	0.006
Ho-proline	0.093	0.006
Methonine	0.297	0.006
Valine	1.413	0.021
Phenylalanine	1.64	0.006
Isoleucine	1.177	0.006
Leucine	1.96	0.010
Histidine	0.716	0.006
Lysine	1.637	0.006
Cysteine	0.01	0.000
Tryptophan	0.486	0.001

Source: (Busani, MORINGA, Patrick, J. MORINGA, Arnold, H. and Voster, MORINGA (2011)

Moringa is reported to not only be protein rich but to have 'high quality protein' which is easily digested and is therefore quickly and easily used by the body. In one 2012 study conducted in India, the dried moringa leaves contained 19 amino acids, which slightly differ from the findings of a 2001 study and a 2009 study which reported 18 and 16 amino acids respectively. The different amounts are attributed to the quality of the growing conditions.

Methionine and cysteine, powerful antioxidants that help in the detoxification of harmful compounds and protect the body from radiation were reported in high concentration in all three studies.

Mineral contents of dried Moringa Oleifera leaves

Mineral	Dry leaf	Standard error
Macro-elements (%)		
Calcium (%)	3.65	0.036
Phosphorous (%)	0.30	0.004
Magnesium (%)	0.50	0.005
Potassium (%)	1.50	0.019
Sodium (%)	0.164	0.017
Sulphur (%)	0.63	0.146
Micro elements (mg/kg)		
Zinc (mg/kg)	31.03	3.410
Copper (mg/kg)	8.25	0.143
Manganese (mg/kg)	86.8	3.940
Iron (mg/kg)	490	49.645
Selenium (mg/kg)	363.00	0.413
Boron (mg/kg)	49.93	2.302

Source: (Busani, MORINGA, Patrick, J. MORINGA, Arnold, H. and Voster, MORINGA (2011)

All of the findings from these many research studies demonstrates that the dry leaves could serve as a protein supplementary source in animal and human diets. This protein content is of particular nutritional significance since it has been suggested that amino acid supplementation is important in meeting a substantial proportion of an animal protein and energy requirements. It is also of remarkable interest that the dried Moringa leaves have been found to have a high deposit of mineral elements. Calcium, for example, was observed to be two to four times higher compared with other plant sources. Calcium, of course, is required for formation and maintenance of healthy bones and teeth thus, preventing osteoporosis. It is also needed for normal blood clothing and nervous functions as well.

Interestingly, even iron, which is commonly deficient in many plant-based diets, was found in abundance in this plant's leaves! As modern science has proven iron is a necessary component of hemoglobin and myoglobin for oxygen transport and cellular processes of growth and division). The presence of zinc in high amounts is of special interest in view of the importance of the inclusion of zinc in the diet of animals and humans. Zinc is also required for cell reproduction and the proper formation of sperm cells. In addition, Zinc is known for its antiviral, anti-bacterial, anti-fungal and anti-cancer properties.

The dried leaves of Moringa also were found to contain copper, which is known to have strong effects on the immune system in general; copper is involved in stimulating body defense systems, as it is active in neutrophil production and affects phagocyte killing ability. It is required for antibody development and lymphocyte killing ability. It is also required for antibody development and lymphocyte replication. Moringa has sulfur which is necessary for efficiency of rumen microbial growth and activity. The dried powdered Moringa leaves have high levels of Vitamin E and beta carotene. Moringa powder has been reported to be rich in beta-caroline, thiamine, riboflavin, niacin, pyrodixine, biotin, ascorbic acid, cholecalciferol, tocophenol and Vitamin K. Beta-carotene rich Moringa leaves can thus be an important sources of vitamin A, can be used for releasing the bound iron status and thus, help in reducing anaemia as well as prevalence of Vitamin A deficiency. Moringa powder is, by the way, so rich in vitamins that it is noted as one of the richest plant sources of vitamins ever discovered.

In a nutshell, the data derived from nutrient characterization of Moringa Oleifera is clear that the plant leaves are rich in a great many nutrients and therefore has the promise and potential to be used as both a feed and food additive with multiple purposes. These include serving as a protein, fatty acid, mineral and vitamin resources for animal and human feed and food formulation. Drying the leaves assists in concentrating the nutrients, facilitates conservation and consumption, and as such, it can be used during any time when feed or food is scarce or it can be easily transported to areas where it is not cultivated at all! Many suggest that Moringa should be consumed in powdered form as its inclusion in the diets could function as a curative, preventative, and therapeutic application.

VITAMIN CONTENT OF MORINGA OLEIFERA

Moringa Oleifera is rich with diverse vitamins, minerals and amino acids. Best of all, these nutrients are readily available for your body use. The great majority of multivitamins available in the supermarket today are created in laboratories, where ingredients are synthesized and packed into a small pill. **Unfortunately, most of these ingredients are not easily absorbed by the body because they are not sourced from whole foods.**

Moringa is a natural, whole food source for vitamins, minerals, proteins, phytonutrients, antioxidants and other important compounds that your body relies on to stay healthy. A single capsule of pure ground moringa, for example, contains a full spectrum of nutrients that are ready for the human body to absorb.

Moringa's benefits are derived from the plant's high concentration of bio-available nutrients. It contains high levels of …

- **<u>VITAMIN A</u>** (beta carotene) is needed by the retina of the eye in the form of a specific metabolite, the light absorbing molecule retinal. This molecule is absolutely necessary for both scotopic vision and color vision. Vitamin A also functions in a very different role as an irreversible oxidized form retinoic acid, which is an important hormone-like growth factor for epithelial and other cells. It is believed that vitamin A is the most important vitamin for immune protection against all kinds of infections. It is involved in healing and bone development. Beta-carotene guards against heart diseases and can keep harmful lipoproteins containing cholesterol from damaging the heart and coronary arteries. It also helps to prevent certain types of cancers and stroke.
- **<u>VITAMIN B1</u>** (thiamine): helps fuel the body by converting blood sugar into energy. It keeps the mucous membrances healthy and is essential for the nervous system and cardiovascular and muscular functions. Moringa leaves contain high amounts of vitamins B1 even compared with the best sources already known. It is higher than green peas, black beans (boiled) and corn (boiled). Vitamin b1 is vital for the production of energy in each cell and it plays an essential role in the metabolism of various carbohydrates.
- **<u>VITAMIN B2</u>** (riboflavin) is required for a wide variety of cellular processes. Like the other B vitamins, it plays a key role in energy metabolism and of the metabolism of fats, ketone bodies, carbohydrates and proteins. It is the central

component of the cofactor FAD and FMN, and is therefore required by all 'flavoproteins'. It is needed to activate viamin B6 and assist the adrenal glands. It is important for red blood cell formation antibody production and growth. It is required for healthy mucous membranes, skin and for the absorption of iron and certain vitamins.

- **VITAMIN B3** (niacin): Like all B complex vitamins is necessary for healthy skin, hair, eyes and liver. It also helps the nervous system function properly. Niacin helps the body produce sex and stress related hormones in the adrenal glands and other parts of the body. It is effective in improving circultation and reducing cholesterol levels in the blood. Moringa leaves and pods contain about 0.5 to 0.8 mg of vitamin B3 per 100 grams (about 3 ounces of vitamin B3 is important for energy production and metabolism of protein, fats and carbohydrates. It supports the function of the digestive system and promotes healthy skin and nerves.

- **VITAMIN B6** (pyridoxine): is required for the synthesis of the neurotransmitters serotonin and norepinephrin and for myelin formation pyridoxine deficiency in adults principally affects the peripheral nerves, skin, mucous membranes and the blood cell systeMoringa

- **VITAMIN B7** (biotin): has vital metabolic functions. Without biotin as a co-factor, many enzymes do not work properly and serious complications can occur, including varied diseases of the skin, intestinal tract and nervous systeMoringa Biotin can help address high blood glucose levels in people with type 2 diabetes and is helpful in maintaining healthy hair and nails, decreasing insulin resistance and improving glucose tolerance and possibly preventing birth defects. It plays a role in energy metabolism and has been used to treat alopecia, cancer, crohn's disease etc.

- **VITAMIN C** (ascorbic acid): just one ounce of moringa leaves contain the daily recommended amount of vitamin C (60mg). In fact, it is so rich in vitamin C that ounce per ounce, it contains 6-7 times that found in orange juice. Vitamin C strengthens our immune system and fight infectious disease including colds & flu, protects against cardiovascular disease, prenatal health problems, eye disease and wrinkles.
- **VITAMIN D** (cholecalciferol): is essential for promoting calcium absorption in the gut and maintaining adequate serum calcium and phosphate concentrations to enable normal mineralization of bone and prevent hypocalcaemia telany. Vitamin D sufficiency prevents rickets in children and osteomalacia in adults. Vitamin D has other roles in human health, including modulation of neuromuscular and immune function and reduction of inflammation.
- **VITAMIN E:** moringa contains large amounts of vitamin E, at 113 mg per 10g (about 3 oz) of the dried leaf powder. The recommended daily intake of vitamin E is 10mg. Vitamin E is a potent antioxidant that helps prevent premature aging and degenerative disease including heart disease, arthritis, diabetes and cancer. It is also known for protecting the body from pollution, increases stamina and reduces or prevents hot flashes in menopause. It promotes younger looking skin, as well as healing and reducing scar tissue from forming.
- **VITAMIN K:** is needed for blood to properly clot and for the liver to make blood clotting factors, including factor II (prothrombin), factor vii (proconvertin), factor ix (thrombiplastin component) and factor x (stuart factor). Other clotting factors that depend on vitamin k are protein C, protein S and protein Z.

NUTRITIVE USES OF MORINGA OLEIFERA

Moringa Oleifera is the most nutrient–rich plant yet discovered. This humble plant has been making strides in less-developed societies for 1000s of years and significant nutritional research has been conducted since the 1970s.

Moringa provides a rich and rare combination of nutrients, amino acids, phytonutrients, antioxidants, antiaging and anti-inflammatory properties used for nutrition and healing. Moringa is sometimes called "mother's best friend' and 'the miracle tree', Moringa has been used for centuries as a reliable source of plant material for nutritional as well medicinal purposes.

These purposes include vitamin C, which fights a host of illnesses including cold and flu, vitamin A, which acts as a shield against eye diseases, skin disease, heart ailments, diarrhea and many other diseases. Calcium, which builds strong bones, and teeth and helps prevent osteoporosis, potassium, which is essential for the functioning of the brain and nerves and proteins, the basic building blocks of all our body cells. Moringa even contains arginine and histidine, two amino acids especially important for infants who are unable to make enough protein for their growth requirement.

It may be useful here to look at each part of the Miracle Tree on its own and note its own health and culinary merits:

- **POD**: the moringa fruit is a long thin pod resembling a drumstick. It is used to prepare a variety of sambar (Sambar is usually a lentil-based vegetable stew or chowder based on a broth made with tamarind popular in South Indian and Sri Lankan Tamil cuisines) and is also fried. It is also preserved by canning and then it is often exported worldwide. It can be made into a variety of curry dishes by mixing with coconut, poppy seeds and mustard. It can be boiled until the drumsticks are semi-soft and consumed directly without any extra processing or cooking. It is used in curries, sambars, korma.

- **LEAVES**: The Moringa Oleifera leaves are highly nutritious, being a significant source of beta–carotene, vitamin C, protein, iron and potassium. The leaves are cooked and used like spinach. In addition to being used fresh as a substitute for spinach. Its leaves are commonly dried and crushed into a powder and used in soups and sauces.

- **FLOWER**: The flowers are edible when cooked and are said to taste like mushrooms. The flowers are just full of nutrition! Flowers infused in honey are used as a cough remedy.

- **BEN OIL**: The moringa seeds yield 38-40% edible oil. The refined oil is clear, odorless and resists rancidity at least as well as any other botanical oil. The seed cake remaining after oil extraction may be used as a good fertilizer or as flocculent to purify water. Oil from the seed, called oil of Ben is used for ear ache and in ointments for skin conditions. The oil rubbed on the skin is said to prevent mosquitoes from biting. When burned in a lamp the oil is smokeless.

- **INDUSTRY USES:** the seed oil is used in arts and for lubricating watches and other delicate machinery and useful in the manufacture of perfumes and hair dressing. The pressed cake obtained after oil extraction may be used as a fertilizer. The industrial uses of the drumstick tree include the use of its wood in paper and textiles industries, bark in the tanning industry. The oil from the seeds contain a powerful flocculent of use in clarifying turbid water.

Therapeutic and Preventative Uses of Moringa Oleifera

Leaf, Flower, Seed, Pod, Root, Bark, Gum, Oil

Antimicrobial		**Endocrine Disorders**	
Skin Infection	LF	Diabetes	LP
Syphilis	G	Hypoglycemia	LP
Typhoid	G	Thyroid	L
Urinary Tract	L	Liver/Kidney	LR
Fungal		Gout	RO
Candida Albicans	O	Bladder Infection	OS
Viral		**Digestive Disorders**	
Common Cold	FRB	Colitis	LB
Epstein-Barr	L	Diarrhea	LR
Herpes Simplex	L	Indigestion	B
HIV-Aids	L	Ulcer, Gastritis	LS
Parasites		**Inflammatory**	
Intestinal, Helminths	LFP	Rheumatism	LFSPRG
Trypanosomes	LR	Arthritis, Joint Pain	SP
Other		Edema	R
Bronchitis	L	Lower Back Pain	R
Jaundice	L	**Neurological**	
Throat Infection	L	Epilepsy	RB
Cancer		Anti-Spasmodic	SR
Anti-Tumor	LFSB	Headache	LRBG
Prostate	L	**Reproductive Health**	
Radioprotective	L	Aphrodisiac	RB
Skin	P	Lactation Enhancer	L
Cardiovascular		Prostate Function	O
Hypertension	LP	Birth Control	B
Diuretic	LFRG	**Skin Disorders**	
Cardiotonic	R	Antiseptic	L
High Cholesterol	L	Astringent	R

Phytochemicals are, in the strictest sense of the word,

chemicals produced by plants. Commonly, though, the word refers to only those chemicals which may have an impact on health, or on flavor, texture, smell, or color of the plants, but are not yet required by humans as essential nutrients (according to the government, anyway).

I am here to tell you though that these phytochemicals, called phytonutrients when we consume them, work in the human body to protect us from the ravages of disease, ageing, injury and daily life in the modern world! An examination of the phytochemicals of Moringa species affords the opportunity to examine a range of fairly unique compounds. In particular, this plant family is rich in compounds containing the simple sugar, rhamnose, and it is rich in a fairly unique group of compounds called glucosinolates and isothiocyanates. For example, specific components of Moringa preparations that have been reported to have hypo-tensive, anticancer, and antibacterial activity include:

- 4-(4'-*O*-acetyl-α-L-rhamnopyranosyloxy) benzyl isothiocyanate [1],
- 4-(α-L-rhamnopyranosyloxy) benzyl isothiocy- anate [2],
- niazimicin [3],
- pterygospermin [4],
- benzyl isothiocyanate [5],
- 4-(α-L-rhamnopyranosyloxy) benzyl glucosinolate [6]
  (Note: numbers after compound refer to picture on next page)

While these compounds are relatively unique to the Moringa family, it is also rich in a number of vitamins and minerals as well as other more commonly recognized phytochemicals such as the carotenoids (including β-carotene or pro-vitamin A).

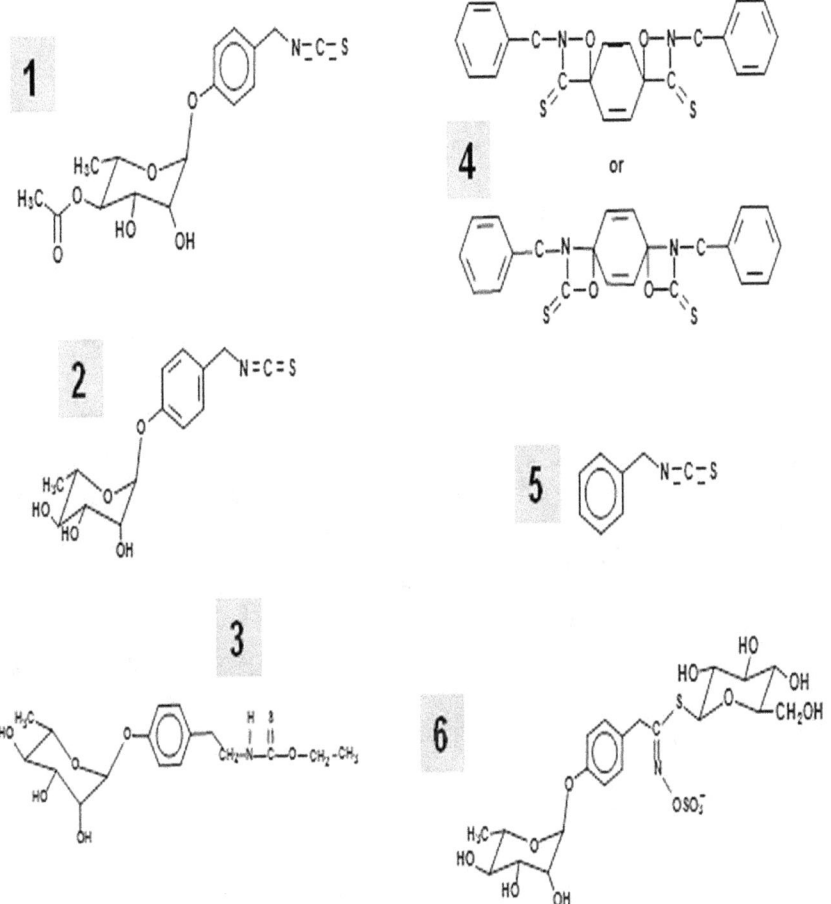

Figure 1. Structures of selected phytochemicals from Moringa spp.: 4-(4'-O-acetyl-α-L-rhamnopyranosyloxy)benzyl isothiocyanate [1], 4-(-L-rhamnopyranosyloxy)benzyl isothiocyanate [2], niazimicin [3], pterygospermin [4], benzyl isothiocyanate [5], and 4-(α-L-rhamnopyranosyloxy)benzyl glucosinolate [6]

6 MORINGA AND...

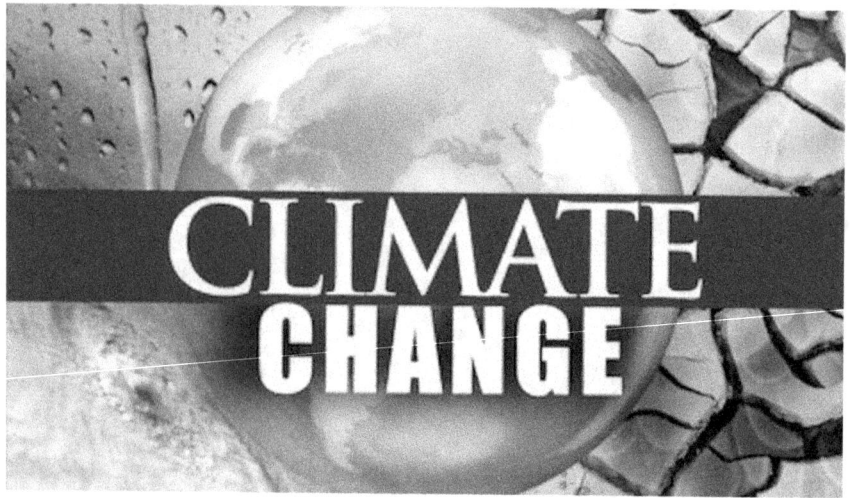

Moringa's Potentials for Climate Change Mitigation

There once was a time in human history when we used tens of thousands of vegetables, cereals, etc. but today we only rely on just a few. What's more, grains may be the most diminished of all. After roughly 10,000 years and 400 generations of progressive agricultural civilization, 70% of the world's food supply comes from just three grains, those being corn, wheat, and rice. Globalization, intensification, and industrialization of agriculture, has been blamed for this trend where we concentrate on very small number of species grown with monoculture farming techniques. Thus global agriculture is leaning too heavily on a few crops and needs to plant a wider variety of crops to build a more resilient food system. The Food and Agriculture Organization of the United Nations (the FAO) reports that crop agriculture is responsible for 14% of global greenhouse gas emissions. Therefore, new climate-smart policies aimed at improving the livelihood of farmers, food security, and food access, as well as reducing emissions of greenhouse gases are the need of the hour.

Climate change, Poverty and Sustainable livelihoods

Sub-Saharan Africa with a population of around 782 million people in 47 nation states is home to 36 of the world's poorest countries. Two-thirds of the estimated 33 million people suffering from AIDS live in sub-Saharan Africa; the region with the highest rates of malnutrition. 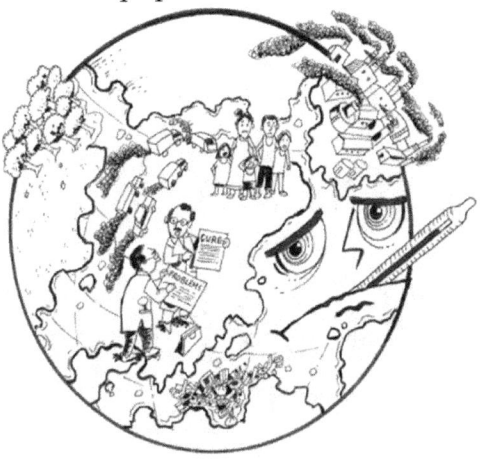 Coincidence? I really can't say but it seems odd to me.

Sub-Saharan Africa is the only major region in the world that has failed to progress in terms of food security with more or less stagnant levels of production per capita in the last 50 years. Climate change presents a new major concern, often interacting with or aggravating existing problems. Small scale farmers in West Africa are already producing far below their potential and since poverty is a rural phenomenon in this region, it is, therefore, only agriculture that holds the key to resolving this problem. As climate change takes firmer hold and the global population grows and the market fluctuates, we need to find ways of resisting the shocks associated with it in order to avoid making an already fragile situation much worse.

Tea, coffee, and cocoa are the three major beverages in the world today. Cocoa was introduced into West Africa about one hundred years ago, and today it is a 50 billion Dollar industry. In Ghana alone cocoa covers 1.8 million hectares. However:

> *"by the year 2080, cocoa, which is Ghana's main export crop, may cease to grow in the country as a result of Climate changes"*

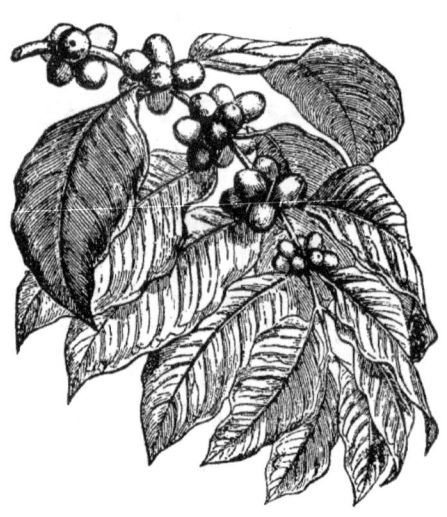

This according to Dr. Raul Gyan of Texas A&M University.

In fact, according to a study by researchers from the Kew Royal Botanic Gardens published in PLoS (The Public Library of Science), the wild Arabica coffee plant, which is the parent of the bushes on nearly all coffee farms the world over, could go extinct as soon as 2080. In China alone tea plantations cover a total of 1.7 million hectares and are the main income of some 80 million farmers. It is needless to say that much of this vegetation and industry is at risk due to Climate change. The environmental impacts caused by human industry are compromising the sustainability of current economic activities, and degrading the natural life support systems, on which we and all other species depend.

Do not get me wrong here, I am not blaming 100% of climate change on human activity alone. Much research has been done which confirms that the planet cycles from cooler to warmer and back again over and over, but to deny that we have any impact at all is tantamount to putting your head in the sand! We must accept our share of the blame and work to correct this!

Climate change is expected to trigger severe consequences to smallholder, poor farmers who dominate the agriculture sector in Africa and much of the developing world. The impacts of climate change are felt at the level of natural resource bases upon which nearly all rural communities depend, at the farming system level and at the level of individual species. Farmers will therefore need to devise mechanisms and adaptation strategies to reduce the impacts of climate change.

Moringa's Potentials and Climate Change

In an independent laboratory test, Moringa Oleifera scored the highest in antioxidant content. Moringa even beat the record-holding acai berry by over a 50% margin, it measured over 157,000 umoles using the Oxygen Radical Absorption Capacity (ORAC) system of measurement developed by the National Institute of Health's National Institute for Aging.

Read that again if you are not completely impressed with Moringa!! The list of antioxidant superfoods used in the research were Moringa, Acai berries, Blueberries, Dark chocolate, Garlic, Goji berries, Green tea, Pomegranates and Red wine. Moringa is naturally vegan, caffeine-free, and gluten-free. The World Health Organization (WHO) and other international humanitarian relief organizations have used Moringa to combat malnutrition in many parts of the world. The many medicinal, nutritional, industrial, and agricultural uses of moringa are well documented.

Dr. Mark Fahey, in a speech to the WHO back in 2005 said that:

> *"the nutritional properties of moringa are now so well known that there seems to be little doubt of the substantial health benefit to be realized by consumption of moringa leaf powder in situations where starvation is imminent."*

The interest generated from the second international conference held in 2006 in Ghana on the uses of the Moringa Tree, has been so great that several national Moringa associations have already been formed in many African countries. Moringa is well adapted to most of sub-Saharan Africa, where the world's worst rates of malnutrition and AIDS are found in spades! Surely that points the way toward solving this human crisis!

The speed with which Moringa Oleifera leaf powder is entering rural markets in Africa is heartening. In Ghana and West Africa, beehives of activities have evolved around Moringa. These offer low cost locally available and sustainable solutions to malnutrition and AIDS support management. The Moringa Tree offers new opportunities to small scale farmers and can contribute to the development of natural resources, but let's not fool ourselves here, it will need strong policies, solid research and savvy market development strategies in order for Moringa to realize its full potential. And what is that potential? **It just may be saving the human race!**

The integration into food systems should be both lateral within Africa and vertical as product development, coupled with market development and penetration efforts, to facilitate the entry of Moringa products into both the developed countries and emerging economic markets.

All of this should be carried out in a way that serves the fundamental interests of all stakeholders, with the most important consideration given to the vulnerable, poor, rural communities wherein primary production occurs. A dynamic new suite of bio-products can be produced from agro-forestry systems that will at the same time contribute to the restoration of badly degraded ecosystems and agricultural site productivity.

When it comes to Global Warming, one practical step to compensate for the several unpreventable carbon dioxide emissions caused by human life and advancement is to plant trees. This is because trees take carbon dioxide (a powerful greenhouse gas) out of the atmosphere and they release oxygen in return. The type of trees planted will have a great influence on the environmental outcome. According to a Japanese study (Villafuerte, and Villafurte-Abonal, 2009) the rate of absorption or assimilation of carbon dioxide by the Moringa tree is twenty times (20x) higher than that of general vegetation and fifty times (50x) higher when compared to the Japanese Cedar Tree (The Japanese Cedar Tree, used in the study, is equivalent to American Cedar Trees in respect to absorption and assimilation of carbon dioxide and the output of oxygen). **This is truly astounding!**

Basically what we learn here is that the Moringa tree can be, and should be, a useful tool in the prevention of Global Warming in that just one single Moringa tree will be equivalent to the effectiveness of fifty (that's right 50!) cedar trees in absorbing carbon dioxide! So, for example, if we expanded the Moringa tree from its current one hundred thousand (100,000) worldwide hectares to (a reasonably achievable) one million (1,000,000) hectares, that would equate to five (5) gigatons of CO_2 being sequestered, that is to say removed or eliminated! Studying how the demand for other superfoods took their rightful positions in the world markets should help product developers to come up with plans, policies and programs to greatly drive demand for their Moringa products in all markets – thus helping the entire planet to heal!

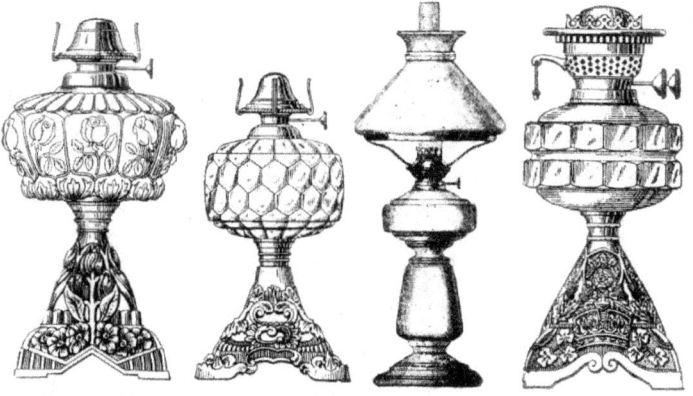

Moringa seeds contain between 30-40% oil, with 13% saturate fats and 82% unsaturated fatty acids. About 65-73% of Moringa oil is oleic acid with olive and sunflower oils having 75% and 40% respectively. Just like olive oil, Moringa oil contains 1-2% of beneficial essential fatty acids such as omega 3 and omega 6. The oil can be used for cooking, as lubricant in fine machinery and as fuel for lamps and in the manufacture of soaps, perfume and hair care products. The seeds and seedcake of Moringa Oleifera are recognized as effective primary coagulant in water treatment as they have the capacity to remove up to 99% of bacteria from water. (See chapter 8 for more on this).

Fresh moringa leaves can be cooked and eaten as vegetables or processed into tea, powder, and other pharmaceutical preparations. Moringa leaves, shoots and seeds can be used as green teas or animal feed with tremendous results. A juice can be extracted from the fresh leaves which can be used as a growth hormone that can increase yields of crops in the field by 25-35% as shown by a study conducted by the University of Bern, in Switzerland.

Moringa is thus a multipurpose plant that is difficult to overlook in today's battle with the climate. It is fast growing and well adapted to growing in adverse conditions where many plants would not be able to, requiring at least 15 ½ inches (400mm) of rain per year. It presents itself as an easy plant for agri-business, poverty mitigation and a climate smart choice of plant to be developed for the benefit of present and future generations. Get on (or two or three) planted today!

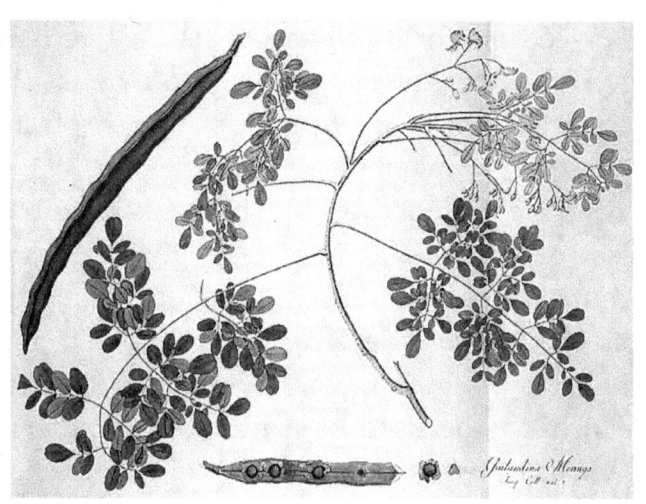

Guilandina Moringa
Coll. vol. 1

68

7   MAKING MORINGA POWDER

Processing the Moringa Leaves into Powder

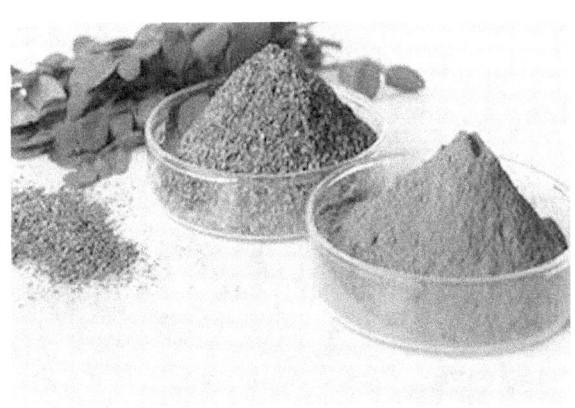 Moringa leaves can be consumed fresh, cooked or dried. Moringa powder is nutritious, easy to make, easy to store and easy to use. Moringa leaf powder is like a multivitamin shot! Powders can be expensive to purchase and quality is always a concern – **Make your own! Moringa leaf powder is the source of incredible health benefits.** There are endless ways to incorporate Moringa Oleifera leaf powder into your diet. Moringa leaf powder can be used as a tea, added to all kinds of drinks and beverages, sprinkled on food or taken in capsules. Moringa powder can be used in cooking or even to top salads. The list of moringa products and ways to apply them is endless!

But Moringa powder is, or can be very expensive, I suggest making your own. It is nothing more than a simple 7 step process:

1.   **Strip the Moringa**
2.   **Wash the Moringa**
3.   **Drain the Moringa**
4.   **Dry the Moringa**
5.   **Mill the Moringa**
6.   **Sieve the Moringa**
7.   **Dry the Powder**

Step 1: Strip the Moringa leaves- Strip all the leaflets from the moringa leaf petiole. This can be done directly from the branches if the moringa leaves have not been stripped off the main branch before transportation. Diseased and damaged leaves are discarded.

Step 2: Washing the Moringa leaves - Wash leaflets in troughs using clean potable water to remove dirt. Wash leaves again in 1% saline solution for 3-5 minutes to remove microbes. Finally wash again in clean water. Leaves are now ready for drying. Drain each trough after each wash: leaves must always be washed with fresh water.

Step 3: Draining the Moringa leaves - Strain the water from the Moringa leaves in buckets that have been perforated, spread leaflets on trays made with food-grade mesh and leave to drain for 15 minutes before taking them to the dryer.

Step 4: Drying the Moringa leaves – Okay, here is where it gets just a bit more involved. There are three main methods for drying moringa leaves:

1.   Room Drying
2.   Solar Drying
3.   Mechanical Drying

Room Drying Moringa leaves:

Spread the moringa leaflets thinly on mesh tied on racks (mosquito net mesh can be used) in a well-ventilated room. This room should be insect, rodent and dust proof. Air circulation can be improved by using ceiling and floor level vents protected with a clean filter to keep the sun and dust out. It is possible to use a fan, but the air must not be directly oriented towards the moringa leaves, as it can increase contamination with germs in the air. It is advisable to turn the moringa leaves over at least once, with sterile gloves, to improve uniform drying. Leaves should be completely dry within a maximum of 4 days. The loading density should not exceed 1 kg/m2.

However, room-dried leaves cannot be guaranteed mold-free with the maximum recommended moisture content of 10%. Therefore, we do not advise this method.

Solar Drying Moringa leaves: If using a commercial solar dryer follow manufactures instructions. In most cases, for best results, spread the leaves thinly on mesh and dry in the dryer for about 4 hours (Temperature range is 95°F–130°F or 35°C–55°C on a very sunny day). The final product should be very brittle.

Mechanical drying Moringa leaves: Use electric or gas hot-air dryers, follow manufactures instructions carefully for best results. Drying temperatures should range between 120°F-130°F (50°C and 55°C). The Moringa leaves should be dried until their moisture content is below 10%.

Step 5: Milling the Moringa Leaves - Mill dry leaves using a stainless steel hammer mill. The leaves can be pounded in a mortar, or milled with a kitchen blender as well. Small-scale processors can use a burr mill or rent a commercial hammer mill for routine milling of their products.

Step 6: Sieving the Moringa Powder - Sieve the Moringa leaf powder if need be. When you mill with a hammer mill, the fineness of the product will depend on the size of the screen used in milling. If too coarse, sift using a sifter with the desired screen size.

Recommended Moringa powder particle sizes are:
- Coarse (1.0 mm – 1.5 mm)
- Fine (0.5 mm – 1.0 mm)
- Very fine (0.2 mm – 0.5 mm)

Step 7: Drying the Moringa leaf powder - Moringa leaf powder strongly attracts moisture and the product can reabsorb humidity during or after milling. for this reason, moringa leaf powder should be dried at 50ºc for 30 minutes to reduce moisture content considerably below 7.5%

Done!!

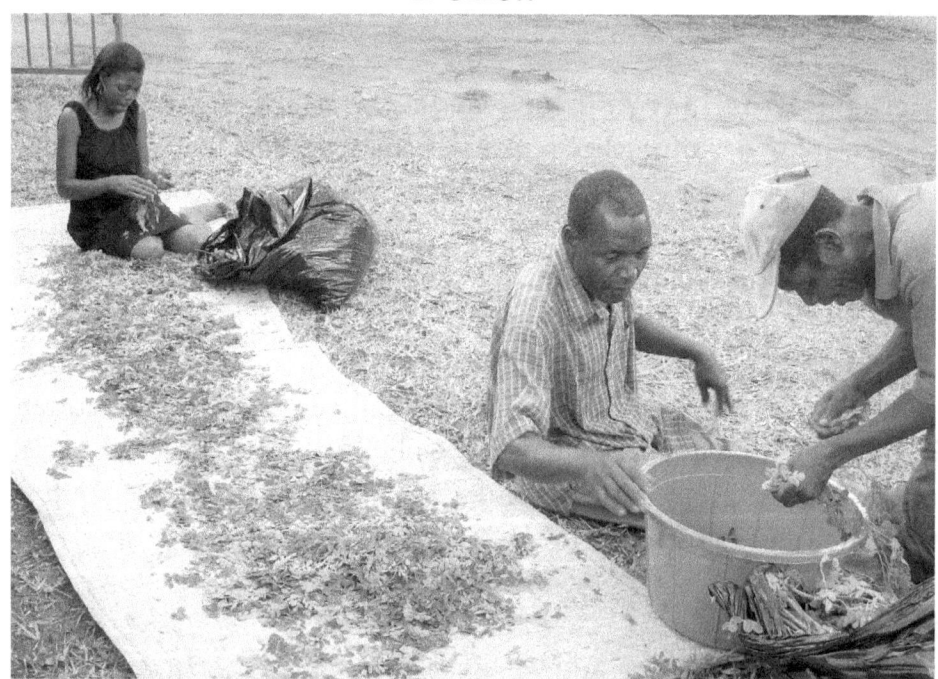

8 HOW TO PURIFY WATER WITH MORINGA SEEDS

Simple Moringa Water Purification Introduction

In addition to food, shelter and clothing, water is one of our basic human needs and lack of potable water is a major cause of death and disease in our world. **<u>Moringa tree to the rescue!</u>**

The Moringa Oleifera seed contains 40% oil by weight, with the remaining presscake containing the active ingredients for natural coagulation. The high market value for the oil makes the case for promoting the cultivation of the seed a strong one. The growth of Moringa Oleifera trees by smallholder farmers should be actively promoted as a means of providing vegetables and raw material for oil extraction in addition to a simple, but effective natural coagulant for turbid river water purification. Yes! Clean water thanks to Moringa oil production!

Using natural materials to clarify water is a technique that has been practiced for centuries and of all the materials that have been used, seeds of the Moringa have been found to be one of the most effective. Studies have been conducted since way back in the early 1970's to test the effectiveness of Moringa seeds for treating water.

These studies confirmed that the seeds are highly effective in removing suspended particles from water with medium to high levels of turbidity. Turbidity is caused by particles suspended or dissolved in water that scatter light making the water appear cloudy or murky. Particulate matter can include sediment - especially clay and silt, fine organic and inorganic matter, soluble colored organic compounds, algae, and other microscopic organisms. (Moringa seeds are less effective at treating water with low levels of turbidity).

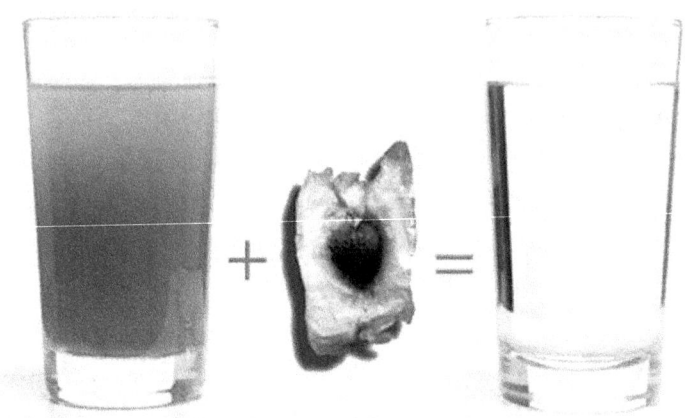

Dirty Water + Moringa Seeds Powder = Clean Water

Moringa Water Purification Theory

Moringa Oleifera seeds treat water on two levels, acting both as a coagulant and an antimicrobial agent. It is generally accepted that Moringa works as a coagulant due to positively charged, water-soluble proteins, which bind with negatively charged particles (silt, clay, bacteria, toxins, etc.) allowing the resulting "flocs" to settle to the bottom or be removed by filtration. The antimicrobial aspects of Moringa continue to be researched. Findings support recombinant proteins both removing microorganisms by coagulation as well as acting directly as growth inhibitors of the microorganisms. While there is ongoing research being conducted on the nature and characteristics of these components, it is accepted by all parties that treatments with Moringa solutions will remove anywhere from 90% up to 99.9% of the impurities in water.

Water Treatment with Moringa Seeds

Solutions of Moringa seeds for water treatment may be prepared from seed kernels or from the solid residue left over after oil extraction (presscake). Moringa seeds, seed kernels or dried presscake can be stored for long periods but Moringa solutions for treating water should be prepared fresh each time. In general, 1 seed kernel will treat 1 litre (1.056 qt.) of water.

Dosage Rates:
- Low turbidity NTU<50 1 seed per 4 liters (4.225 qt) water
- Medium turbidity NTU 50-150 1 seed per 2 liters (2.112 qt) water
- High turbidity NTU 150-250 1 seed per 1 liter (1.056 qt) water
- Extreme turbidity NTU >250 2 seeds per 1 liter (1.056 qt) water

INSTRUCTIONS TO CLEAN WATER WITH MORINGA SEEDS

1. Collect mature *Moringa Oleifera* seed pods and remove seeds from pods.
2. Shell seeds (remove seed coat) to obtain clean seed kernels; discard any discolored seeds.
3. Determine quantity of kernels needed based on amount and turbidity of water; in general, 1 seed kernel will treat 1 litre (1.056 qt.) of water.

4. Crush appropriate number of seed kernels (using grinder, mortar & pestle, etc.) to obtain a fine powder and sift the powder through a screen or small mesh.
5. Mix seed powder with a small amount of clean water to form a paste.
6. Mix the paste and 250 ml (1 cup) of clean water into a bottle and shake for 1 minute to activate the coagulant properties and form a solution.
7. Filter this solution through a muslin cloth or fine mesh screen (to remove insoluble materials) and into the water to be treated.
8. Stir treated water rapidly for at least 1 minute then slowly (15-20 rotations per minute) for 5-10 minutes.
9. Let the treated water sit without disturbing for at least 1-2 hours.
10. When the particles and contaminates have settled to the bottom, the clean water can be carefully poured off.
11. This clean water can then be filtered or sterilized to make it completely safe for drinking.

DANGERS

Secondary Infection: The process of shaking and stirring must be followed closely to activate the coagulant properties; if the flocculation process takes too long, there is a risk of secondary bacteria growth.

Recontamination: The process of settling is important. The sediment at the bottom contains the impurities so care must be taken to use only the clear water off the top and not allow the sediment to re-contaminate the cleared water.

Additional contaminants: Moringa treatment does not remove 100% of water pathogens.

Using Moringa Oleifera as a replacement coagulant for proprietary coagulants meets the need for water and wastewater technology in developing countries which is simple to use, robust and cheap to both install and maintain. Water purified with Moringa seeds, is acceptable for drinking only in serious emergencies of imminent dehydration or in areas where people are currently drinking untreated, contaminated water.

How to Purify Water with Moringa Seeds

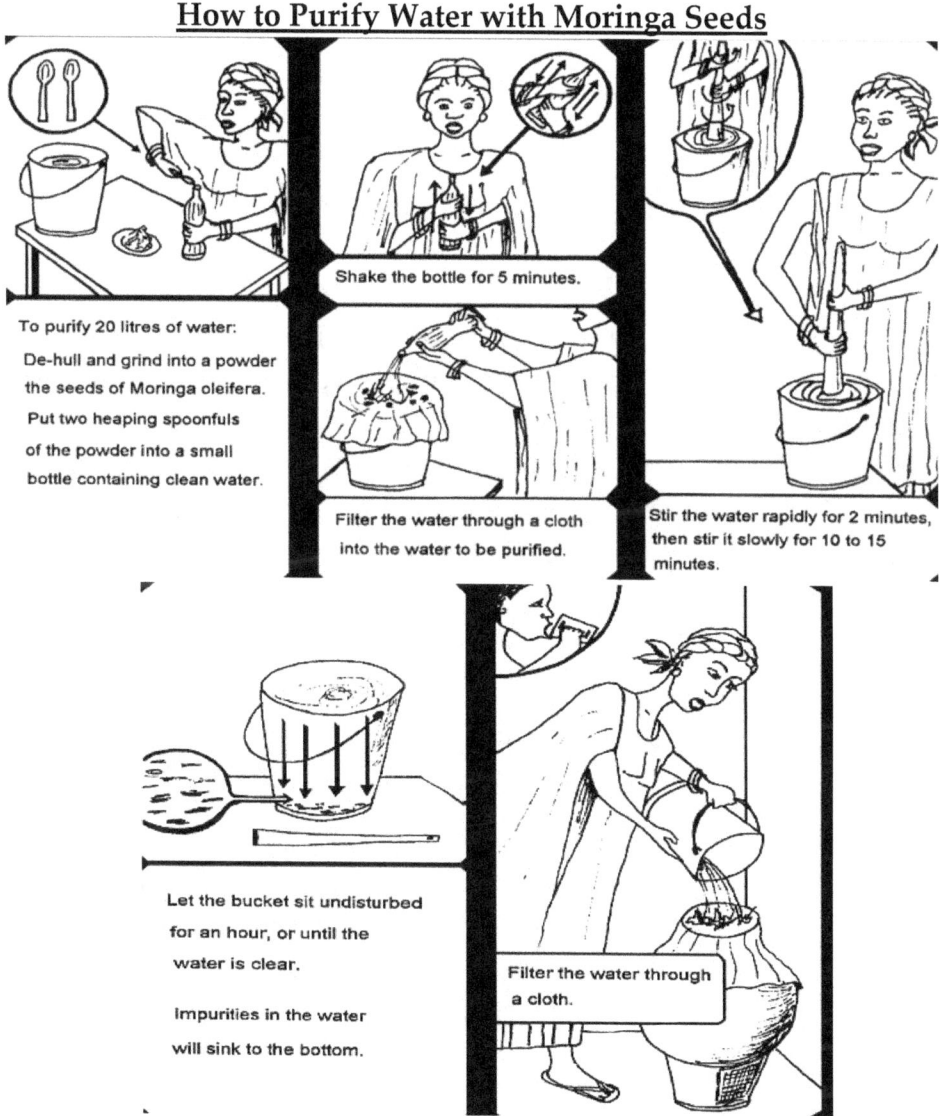

To purify 20 litres of water:

De-hull and grind into a powder the seeds of Moringa oleifera. Put two heaping spoonfuls of the powder into a small bottle containing clean water.

Shake the bottle for 5 minutes.

Filter the water through a cloth into the water to be purified.

Stir the water rapidly for 2 minutes, then stir it slowly for 10 to 15 minutes.

Let the bucket sit undisturbed for an hour, or until the water is clear.

Impurities in the water will sink to the bottom.

Filter the water through a cloth.

9   MAKING MORINGA TEA

Moringa Oleifera tea is an excellent energy drink. The tea is loaded with antioxidants and vitamins that will help clear your mind and boost your energy levels. You can prepare a tea by steeping a handful of dry leaves in hot water for a few minutes. Dried Moringa leaf tea creates a refreshing and nutritious energy boost you will really come to appreciate.

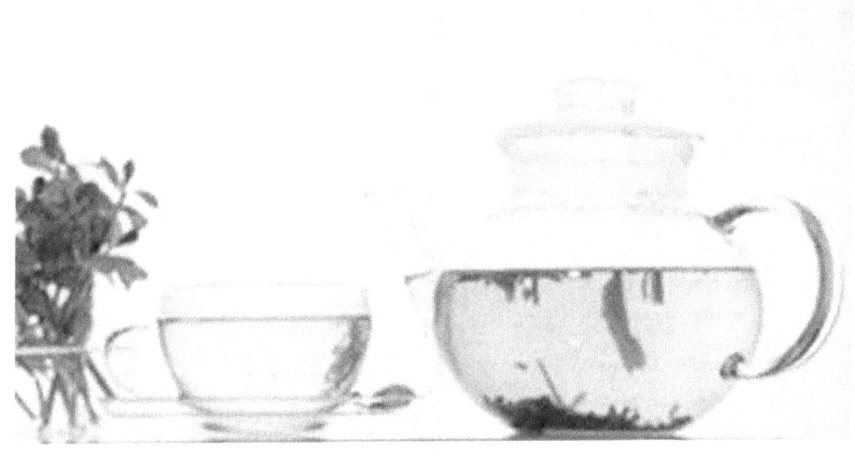

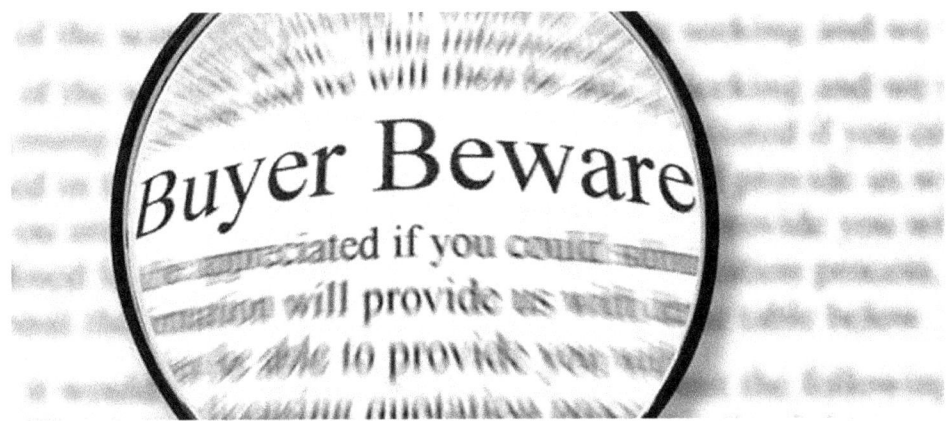

If you choose to purchase Moringa Tea be very sure you are getting tea that comes from 100% Pure Moringa Oleifera, not all companies sell 100% Moringa Oleifera!

What makes Moringa Oleifera tea so healthy and delicious? It is all-natural, energy packed like no other tea. In fact, it is not a tea at all. All teas are derived from the Camellia sinensis plant. Moringa tea is actually a tisane and unlike tea, contains no caffeine at all.

An Antioxidant-Rich Energy Booster

Moringa Oleifera is one of the richest sources of nutrients and vitamins that our body needs. Moringa can be prepared as a vegetable or included in soups, but mostly just the leaves and fruits are used. Others prefer to drink it as tea.

Here are some simple steps on how to make Moringa tea and Moringa powder.

To make Moringa tea you should harvest fresh leaves from your tree and dry them at room temperature. Place the leaves in a brown paper bag with some holes in it and hang the bag in a cool area of your home. In about 10-14 days your leaves should be dry enough to use. To make the tea, shred or pulverize the leaves.

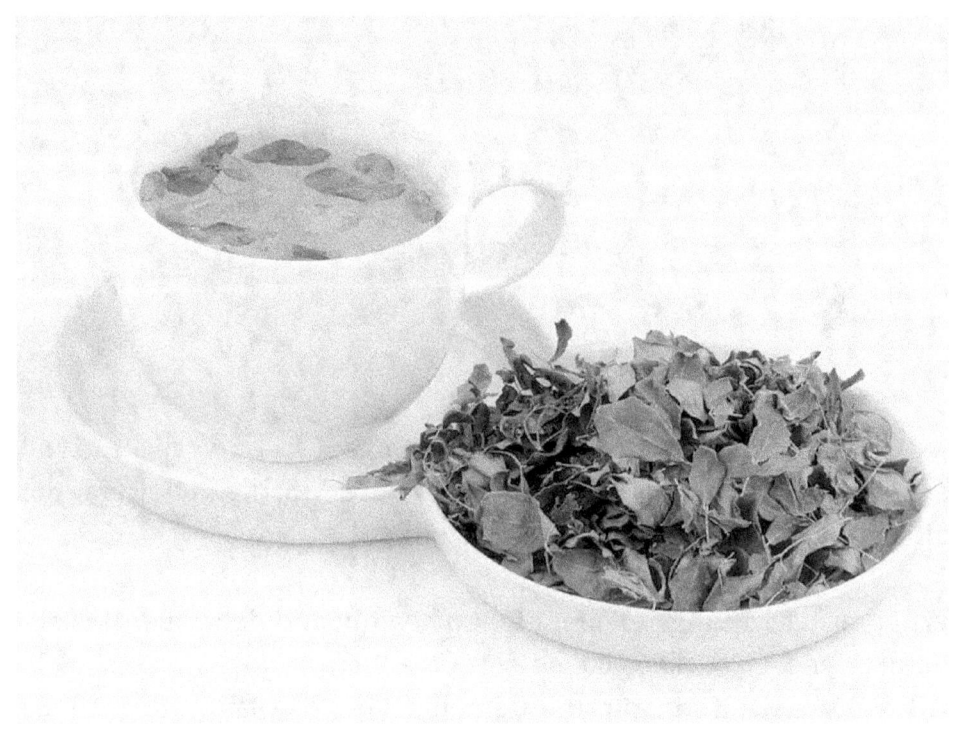

Every cup of tea you drink will provide you with vital nutrients. Moringa tea is well respected and known to be an excellent defense against damaging free radicals.

Moringa Hot Tea Recipe #1

<u>Step 1 - Get Moringa Leaves -</u> Gather Moringa leaves, 3 to 4 stalks will do. It is best to use the mature leaves because they dry up fast.

<u>Moringa Tea Step 2 - Air Drying -</u> Air dry the leaves including the stalks for a day or until the leaves are crisp. Air drying will make the leaves fall out and then you can separate the stalks after. But some people include the stalk in making tea because of its fiber content.

Moringa Tea Step 3 – Grinding - Grind the air-dried leaves (with the stalks if you prefer) for 10-15 seconds. You can use a blender to grind the leaves.

Moringa Tea Step 4 – Storage - Put the ground Moringa in tea bags, and store in a cool, dry place. Make sure not to leave it in open moist places, so it will have a long shelf-life.

Moringa Tea Step 5 - Preparing the Tea - To prepare Moringa tea, just add hot water, lemon and sugar to taste.

Moringa Hot Tea Recipe #2

- You can use your electric coffee maker to make Moringa leaf tea. Here is how to do it. Add the same amount of Moringa leaf to your filter as you would for each cup of coffee you plan to brew. For a single cup use between 1/2 to 1 teaspoon.

Iced Moringa Leaf Tea Recipe

- Add 1- 1/12 teaspoon of Moringa leaf to 16 ounces of water. Mix with a little honey and fresh ginger and orange Juice to taste.
- Blend in your blender or shake vigorously for one minute, add ice and refrigerate for 8 hours.

Moringa Leaf Tea Benefits

There have been many different benefits reported by those who buy organic Moringa and consume it on a daily basis. One benefit is the fact that there is no caffeine present in the drink. Instead those who buy Moringa tea notice that the vitamins help to provide energy to the body, along with a boost in digestion. Throughout time Moringa leaf tea has been used around the world as a great source of needed vitamins, and even has been used to help fight against ailments and illnesses.

Where to Buy Moringa Tea?

When it comes to knowing where to buy Moringa tea, there are a variety of vendors that can be found online. However, it is important to know that not all of those who you can buy organic Moringa from have the best quality product. Before you buy Moringa Oleifera, it is important to look at the history of the provider as well as how they produce their Moringa tea and their experience in the industry.

You can buy Moringa tea as a great first step in the direction of leading a healthy life filled with all of the necessary nutrients, minerals and vitamins your body needs. Buy Moringa Oleifera tea and start feeling the benefits first hand.

Moringa Trumps All Superfood Rivals in ORAC Tests

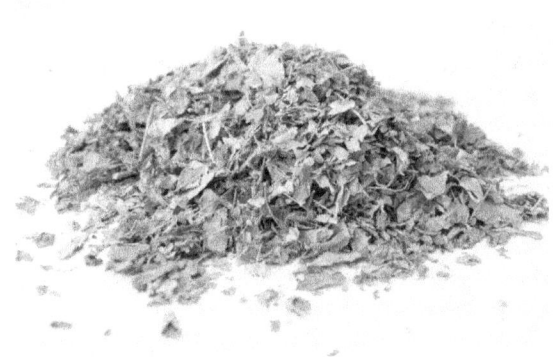

Brunswick Laboratories performed an independent study, (in-vitro) using Moringa leaf tea to test its Oxygen Radical Absorbance Capacity (or ORAC value score). The ORAC value score is the industry accepted measurement of antioxidants in foods and supplements. **Antioxidants** are compounds which actively **quench free-radicals** which helps to prevent cellular damage, a common pathway for cancer, aging and a variety of diseases.

With an amazing score of 157,000 umole TE/100g (*hydrophilic and lipophilic*) Moringa beat out all other antioxidant superfoods, including rivals such as matcha tea at 134,000, turmeric at 127,000 and acai at 102,700. Surprisingly green tea, which is renowned for its antioxidant health benefits could only muster a score of 1, 240.

10   ABOUT MORINGA OIL – NOT JUST A COSMETICS LEGEND!

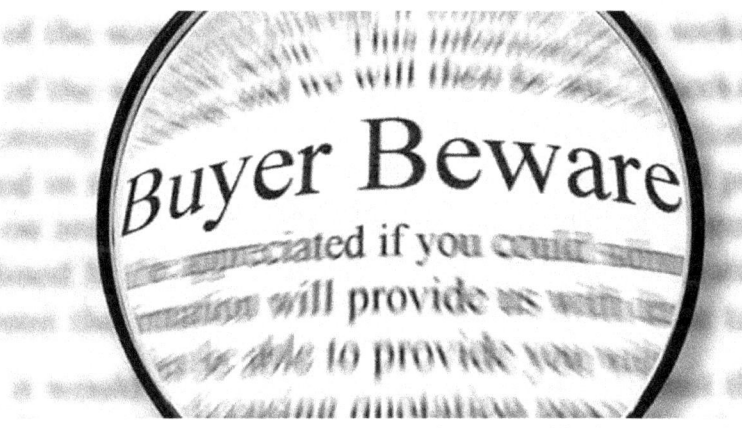

Apparently most Moringa Oil is not the real stuff! Therefore, buyer beware. Moringa oil is 20 times the cost of vegetable oil so the motivation is definitely there for diluting the oil with something cheaper. Research the company you are going to purchase from before you buy.

The natural goodness of Moringa oil dates back thousands of years ago. The Egyptians, the Greeks and then Romans, all recognized the natural properties of Moringa oil and used it extensively in perfumes and as skin softeners. The Egyptians also recognized its natural protective properties and used it on their skin to protect themselves from the harsh desert conditions with which they dealt with on a daily basis. Both of these uses have been documented by these ancient cultures. It is no wonder that modern cosmetic manufacture are beginning to include it in their most expensive products.

Help for dry skin
- It softens dry skin and maintains moisture in the skin.
- It is good for conditioning dry, chapped lips.
- It's beneficial to treat rough, dry skin conditions like dermatitis, eczema and psoriasis.

Anti-aging properties
- Moringa oil rejuvenates dull, tired and aging skin
- Moringa oil antioxidants and nutrients help fight free radical damage that can cause skin tissue damage and lead to the formation of wrinkles
- Moringa oil helps improve the appearance of wrinkles and prevents sagging of facial muscles.
- Moringa oil has hormones called cytokinins, which help promote cell growth and delay damage and destruction of skin tissues.
- Vitamin C stabilizes collagen and helps reduce fine lines and repair damaged skin cells.

Antiseptic and anti-inflammatory properties
- Moringa oil has antiseptic and anti-inflammatory properties and has been used to treat and heal minor skin abrasions; minor cuts and scrapes, bruises, burns, insect bites, rashes, and sunburn and skin infections

Acne & dark spot prevention
- Moringa oil helps clear blackheads and pimples. When used regularly helps prevent the reoccurrence of blemishes

- Helps minimize dark spots caused by acne and hyperpigmentation
- Moringa oil has nourishing and emollient properties giving it benefits for use in skin and hair care products
- Moringa oil is useful in lifting dirt out of the hair and is an efficient natural cleanser. By simply wetting the hair, massaging the oil into the scalp and rinsing can effectively clean and moisturize the scalp
- The Moringa oil does not become rancid for several years after it is produced

Moringa oil is a concentrated source of food energy

Small amounts of Moringa oil added to the diet of young children can provide them with a more varied and nutritious diet. Moringa oil is rich in vitamins and unsaturated fatty acids. Moringa oil contains antiseptic and anti-inflammatory properties, which help heal minor skin complaints such as cuts, bruises, burns, insect bites, rashes and scrapes quickly. Its use can be traced back to the ancient Egyptians, who placed vases filled with moringa oil inside their tombs.

Moringa oil is among the most desired oils to produce skin care products and for cosmetics, because of its various antioxidants and skin rejuvenating qualities. The industry loves this stuff – and so should you! These antioxidants do wonders for aging and skins lucking nutrients.

With a great amount of oleic acid content of 72%, Moringa oil penetrates very deep into the skin, bringing the necessary nutrients to the skin and hair, helping it to retain moisture. Moringa oil can be used to increase the health and strength of the hair and scalp. So one of the greatest advantages of moringa oil, is skin care and rejuvenation, stronger and healthier hair. Although there are new and innovative ways to reduce wrinkles and restore vitality to the skin, the secret to youthful skin lies in keeping a healthy living environment for skin cells to live, and Moringa oil can do this very well.

To enjoy the wonderful benefits of moringa on skin, simply apply moringa oil and lightly massage on skin. Leave it on for several minutes so the skin can be nourished with the vitamins and minerals present in moringa.

Moringa oil can also be applied in the production of expensive and natural perfumes and fragrances. Moringa oil's high oleic level, combined with its enduring shelf life, make it a popular choice for traditional perfume production.

Perfume makers value moringa oil because it has the ability to absorb and retain even the most volatile scents. It has been used in effleurage, a process that uses solid, odorless fats to capture the fragrances of delicate plants and flowers. Effleurage is a traditional method of extracting essential oils from these plants, although it is time-consuming and expensive. Moringa, however, is one of the choice oils for perfume manufacturers that still employ the 'old school' effleurage process.

Because Moringa oil contains powerful antioxidants, it can also be used and included in soaps, shampoos, body washes and skin scrubs. Moringa oil absorbs rapidly into the skin, making it is a good choice for beauty products that are rinsed off the skin, such as soaps and shampoos.

Moringa oil is one of the most exotic and highly searched for oil's around the world.

As awareness arises about moringa you are starting to see it listed in high end cosmetics as an ingredient to help slow the signs of aging and to moisturize. Before you buy, take a look at the rest of the ingredients and the company itself to determine if the moringa contained within will actually be beneficial to you and good for the planet.

Same story for all moringa products is valid. Before you buy a moringa supplement, make sure you do your due diligence on the manufacturer and where they source their moringa from and any other ingredients the products contain.

The Seeds can be extracted and eaten as "peas" (boiled or fried) when still green. The dry seeds are apparently not used for human consumption, perhaps because the bitter coating becomes hardened. Moringa Seeds from mature pods should be roasted, mashed and placed in boiling water for 5 minutes. After straining and sitting overnight, the moringa oil floats to the surface.

Moringa seed has a fairly soft kernel, so the oil can be extracted by hand using a screw press (also known as a "spindle" or "bridge" press). The seed is first crushed, 10% by volume of water is added, followed by gentle heating over a low fire for 10-15 minutes, taking care not to burn the seed. One such test yielded 2.6 liters of oil from 11 kg of kernels. Once the best processing conditions are worked out, an extraction efficiency of 65% could probably be expected.

BIOMASA has also researched moringa seed oil extraction. M. Fuglie, the main researcher states the following in his report:

> "*Nikolaus Foidl designed a motorized moringa seed de-huller with a built-in blower to separate out the chaff. The de-hulling part of the machine consists of two revolving rubber plates slightly oval in shape. Seed is run through 3 times, with the space between the plates diminished slightly each time (smaller seed not de-hulled the first time will be de-hulled the 2nd or 3rd time).*"

Foidl suggests that a screw press made of simple iron may be better suited for moringa oil extraction than one made of steel. Chromium and nickel in steel may react with the oil at high temperatures and lower oil quality.

Fuglie continues,

> *"Following extraction, moringa oil should be filtered (through cheese cloth or coffee filter). This will remove the protein content upon which bacteria feed. Viscosity of oil can be improved by heating it to 40-50 °C before filtering."*

At Church World Service in Senegal, one oil extraction trial used kernels that had been de-hulled three months earlier. The oil promptly separated into a milky wax and liquid. This was probably due to the rapid deterioration in the stored kernels of the antioxidant tocopheral acetate (Vitamin E). A few (1-5) drops per liter of the essential oil of sage, rosemary or mint (or a twig of the latter), all excellent antioxidants themselves, can be added to moringa oil to stabilize it.

The seedcake left over after the oil extraction process has several uses. It can be used as soil fertilizer or in the treatment of turbid water (see chapter 8). It is being researched as an animal feed, but has a bitter taste and contains anti-nutritional factors (such as glucosinolates, haemagglutinins, alkaloids and a saponin). I have read that in order to remove the bitter taste and anti-nutritional factors, you can soak the seedcake in water for 20 to 30 minutes, then sieve it to recover the residue. I do not know of feeding trials that were done in the field to test this method so if you try it let me know how it goes!

In Summary, Moringa Oil or Ben oil is obtained by pressing the seeds of the Moringa Oleifera tree. The Moringa seeds yield

38% to 40% edible oil (called ben oil, from the high concentration of behenic acid contained in the oil) that can be used in cooking, cosmetics, and lubrication.

Traditionally used for cooking and in other food preparations. Moringa oil has tremendous cosmetic value and is used in body and hair care as a moisturizer and skin conditioner. It can be used for perfume base as a fuel and for oiling machinery. Moringa oil can also be used to produce soapMoringa oil is light and spreads easily on the skin. It is best for massage and aromatherapy applications.

Moringa oil is used in the following range of cosmetic products.

- Anti-aging, wrinkle creams
- Hair care products
- Soaps and Liquid body wash
- Aromatherapy oils
- Massage Oils
- Face creams
- Perfumes
- Deodorants

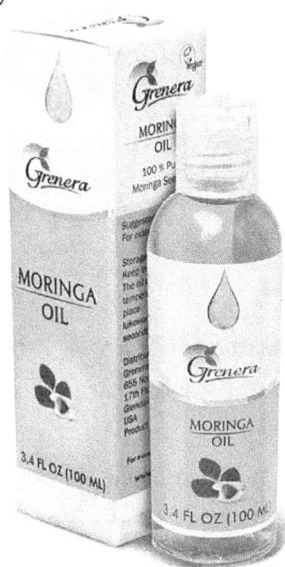

11   MORINGA HISTORY

Moringa Oleifera is beginning to draw lots of attention in scientific circles for its medical and nutritional benefits. Already the Moringa tree is making its way internationally to help resolve starvation issues around the world, standing up as one of the few true "superfoods" in the world. However, the history of Moringa extends back to well before the time when it fell under the scrutiny of Western science. The benefits of Moringa have been known, appreciated and passed down in Asia for many generations; for many centuries. This ancient knowledge has now fallen under the lens of science, and it turns out: the history has a strong case for proving this remarkable tree as a true "lifesaving gift of nature."

History

I want to take a few pages here and look at a bit more at the fascinating history of Moringa. The history of the Moringa tree starts, as best as we can tell, in the southern Himalayas, with roots in India, Pakistan, Bangladesh, and Afghanistan. Although the timber of the drumstick tree was found to be a poor source for construction material or even fires, the tree itself was quickly recognized as a food source. As such, the Romans, Greeks, and

Egyptians all cultivated the Moringa tree as these civilizations entered the regions where the trees grew. From India, it spread to ancient Egypt, where it was used as a natural sunscreen to protect against the harsh desert environment; and then eventually to Greece and Rome where it served an important role as both an ointment and expensive perfume. Soon the prized trees were being sent back to Roman Emperors, Greek Politicians and Egyptian Pharos alike. The progress of the plant also moved westward into Southeast Asia and the Pacific Islands (most notably the Philippines), where its unique nutritional qualities caused it to become a staple vegetable in the local diet. Now we find it moving into western cultures and even into my backyard in Texas.

As I researched Moringa I became interested in the fact that it has been used for centuries as both a food source and a medicine – I wanted to know how far back I could trace its use.

Let us take a quick look in the Bible; in the Bible book of Exodus (15:22-26) it is written:

> [22] So Moses brought Israel from the Red Sea; then they went out into the Wilderness of Shur. And they went three days in the wilderness and found no water. [23] Now when they came to Marah, they could not drink the waters of Marah, for they were bitter. Therefore, the name of it was called Marah. [24] And the people complained against Moses, saying, "What shall we drink?" [25] So he cried out to the LORD, and the LORD showed him a tree. When he cast it into the waters, the waters were made sweet.
> There He made a statute and an ordinance for them, and there He tested them, [26] and said, "If you

diligently heed the voice of the LORD your God and do what is right in His sight, give ear to His commandments and keep all His statutes, I will put none of the diseases on you which I have brought on the Egyptians. For I am the LORD who heals you."

Ok, so after escaping Egypt, Moses and the Israelites were lost in the desert and very thirsty. They eventually found water but it was not good to drink. Then God showed Moses that he could use a tree to make the water safe to drink and God goes on to promise that if the Israelites do as he says he will protect them from all of the diseases which "I have brought on the Egyptians."

That is very interesting, it sounds remarkably like a biblical reference to the moringa tree. I mean, ask yourself, "Are there really trees that can turn bad water into clean drinking water — trees that will purify water quickly to make it drinkable?"

Yes there is, as we discussed in Chapter 8 of this book, Moringa is used, has been used and will continue to be used to help clean and purify water! One of the most remarkably useful trees in the world the Moringa tree is being cultivated heavily for use in the Sudan. The Food and Agriculture Organization of the United Nations has stated that village women had successfully used the tree *Moringa oleifera* to cleanse the highly turbid water of the River Nile. After trying other moringa species in Egypt, Namibia, Somalia, and Kenya, they too have shown properties that clarify water quickly.

I cannot be 100% sure in saying that the moringa was the tree the Israelites used to purify the waters of Marah. The Bible does not give us enough information about either the tree or the water to make that conclusion. Nor is it certain in the passage whether the miracle was in God's revealing to Moses the type of tree that would solve the problem, or in God's producing a one-off miracle using a tree at the campsite. But the wording that says "the Lord shewed him [Moses] a tree" seems to be saying the solution was, in fact, the tree. At least that is the way it seems to me.

Let us, for the sake of argument, assume that the passage above does refer to the Moringa tree, that then would mean that it was in use, in the area of Egypt, over four thousand years ago.

The next question one must answer is, "Are there any other references to the use of Moringa in ancient times?"

Today we know that all parts of the tree are edible, the highest nutritional value comes from consuming the leaves, ideally in a dried and powdered form. While its nutritional benefits are known to us were they known to ancient man? Well, the simple fact that many cultures the world over know about the nutritional and medicinal value of the Moringa – without the benefit of modern science – speaks to the very fact that the ancients did know and were careful to pass on that knowledge to their children and grandchildren. How they knew this is another question altogether but the fact is that many of the benefits of Moringa were known. In fact, it seems that it was quickly discovered by ancient civilizations that the tree also provided many medicinal benefits, most notably an energy boost. Those who used Moringa found themselves experiencing inordinately high amounts of energy when compared to others, and it was believed to have many other medicinal properties as well.

As a consequence of its versatility, the tree has spread far and wide. One of the remarkable properties of the tree is its ability to survive in dry regions (though it is susceptible to the cold), as such it was destined to grow well in Egypt.

Moringa spread east from India to China, Asia, west to Egypt, the Horn of Africa, around the Mediterranean and the West Indies. There has been evidence of its use from 2000 BC on. It was highly valued by the Greeks, Romans and Egyptians alike. The oil, made from the seed, was used as a skin protection against the sun, carrier oil for perfumes and medicines. The seeds were also used for water purification.

A tomb dated from the 18th dynasty (1550-1292 BC) in Egypt was found to contain 10 jars of 'Sweet Moringa oil' thought to have been used in the funeral procession ritual.

In Qasr Ibrim, once a major city in what is now Lake Nasser, traces of Moringa were found to be present as early as the 7th century BC. Forth century BC evidence shows that a base oil made from the seed nut of the Moringa was highly coveted as it was less viscous and very receptive to absorbing scent and its origin was the Syrian and Egyptian desserts.

References in the Bible have also been claimed to pertain to the Moringa tree as we discussed above. But other references exist in the Bible leading may to suggest that the Moringa tree is actually the "Tree of Life" discussed in the Bible.

We saw a possible reference in the book of Exodus above and Studies carried out since the 1970's consistently show crushed Moringa seeds are effective in removing suspended particles with medium to high levels of turbidity (muddiness or dirtiness) from water. Another reference in the Bible that may well refer to the Moringa tree is found in the book of Revelations.

"Then the angel showed me the river of the water
of life, as clear as crystal, flowing from the throne of

God and of the Lamb [2] down the middle of the great street of the city. On each side of the river stood the tree of life, bearing twelve crops of fruit, yielding its fruit every month. **And the leaves of the tree are for the healing of the nations. [3] No longer will there be any curse.** The throne of God and of the Lamb will be in the city, and his servants will serve him.Revelations 22; 1-3

The section of the passage in bold, above is often claimed to be evidence that the Moringa Tree is the Tree of Life. Further, there is also mention of a tree in the Qur'an which has sometimes been thought of as the olive tree but modern thinking goes more towards the Moringa as the seeds contain 40% oil where the olive only 20%.

> "And a tree that springs forth from Mount Sinai, that grows oil and relish for the eaters."
> – Sirah 3 Al-Mu'minun pert 18; 20

Lise Manniche, in 'An Ancient Egyptian Herbal' gives recipes that were used by the ancient Egyptians. It would appear that Moringa oil was used as a carrier oil which would be mixed with various other ingredients for medicinal purposes. For example:
"**Maladies of the stomach** – Moringa oil, honey, frankincense, wine which would be boiled from a paste and eaten.
Cramp – Moringa oil, barley flour, ox fat, boiled and eaten.
Sore gums – Moringa oil, gum, fig, ochre and water rubbed onto gums.
Maladies of the head – Moringa oil, castor oil seeds, fat, made into a poultice and placed on the head.

Poultice to stop bleeding – Moringa oil, wax, fat, honey, carob pulp and boiled barley.

Ear ache – Moringa oil, cucumber, ochre.

Wrinkles – Moringa oil, frankincense gum, wax, cypress grass ground finely with fermented plant juice and applied daily."

What is more, Moringa oil was used on a daily basis as a mosquito repellent. Research conducted in Berlin, Germany in 2012 shows that the Moringa oil, applied to the skin topically does indeed repel those pesky, often disease carrying mosquitos.

Finally, although not in Egypt, a story about the only time Alexander the Great was beaten in battle also mentions moringa use in the ancient world. In India, in 326 BC, over a two-year period and encompassing around sixty battles, Alexander the Great was finally defeated by the Maurian peoples who then carved out an empire that included most of the Indian subcontinent, except for the Tamil-speaking south. It was recorded that these peoples fed on a liquid Moringa diet during their fight against Alexander the Great, and that this gave them almost 'super human' strength as they needed little sleep, they never got sick, their wounds healed rapidly, and in the end, they wore Alexander's army down and crushed it.

It does appear that there is evidence for the use and knowledge of the Moringa tree in ancient times, but is it the 'Tree of Life' mentioned in the Bible? Evidence to make that claim is not as clear:

Trees are significant in biblical symbolism. A study of trees in Genesis helps us to understand the ancient world of Abraham and his Kushite ancestors.

The trees known to have grown in the region of Abraham's people include acacia, cedar, date nut palms, sycamore fig trees and baobab. These figure prominently in biblical symbolism, although not all are mentioned in Genesis. Acacia and cedar were used in the construction of the Ark and the Tabernacle. The baobab tree is likely the origin of the idea of waters flowing from a tree as in Revelation 22:1-2.

Six trees are especially important in the symbolism of Genesis: the Tree of Life; the Tree of the Knowledge of Good and Evil; fruit-bearing trees; the prophet's oak at Mamre, the "trees" used to build Noah's ark, and the date palm (tamar) which grew around water shrines. None of these however is the Moringa tree. But that does not mean that the Tree of Life and the Moringa tree are not one and the same. Let's dig a bit deeper.

The Tree of Life is a very old idea, as is evident from the wide diffusion of the motif across Africa, Asia, Australia and South America. The principle of diffusion holds that the oldest culture traits, beliefs or practices are those that are most widely diffused across the earth. So, we may assume that the Tree of Life motif is indeed very ancient. The Tree of Life archetype is as old as the serpent archetype and the two are often portrayed together, as in the image (below) of Re's cat killing Apophis, the giant water serpent. The point of origin of both archetypes

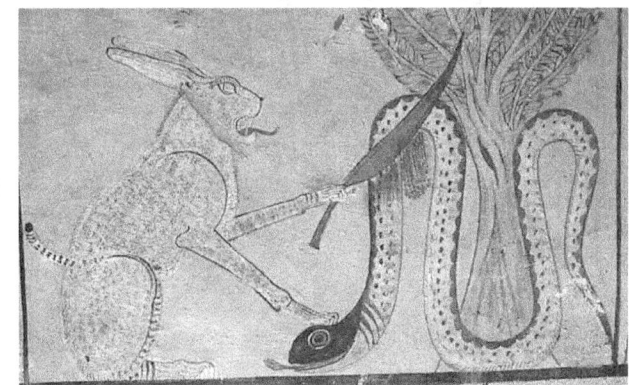

appears to be the Nile.

The Kikuyu, a Nilotic tribe, place their first 'parents' on a ridge north of Muranga, a town south of Nyeri in Kenya. One can still visit the site today. If you do go there, you will notice a sky-blue gate which marks the entrance to Mukurwe Wa Nyagathanga—the Tree of Gathanga. Inside the gate are two mud huts, one for Gikuyu and one for Mumbi. The site looks toward the cloud-shrouded Mount Kenya (called "Mount Kirinyaga" in precolonial times). To the Kikuyu, Mount Kenya is the seat of God, who they call Ngai.

Ngai created Gikuyu and told him: "Build your homestead where the fig trees grow." This is why many believe that the Tree of Life was a fig tree. Genesis does not say what kind of fruit was produced by the Tree of Life, but the fig tree plays a significant role in revealing Jesus as the Son of God in the Gospels (Mark 11, Matthew 21 and Luke 13).

Mount Kenya stands at 15,000 feet and is 42 miles west-southwest of Mount Kilimanjaro. It is an extinct volcanic crater and the land at the base is rich volcanic soil. As one ascends the mountain, there are forests with fig trees.

Among the Christian Church Fathers, the Tree of Life is a symbol of Jesus Christ and the serpent is the symbol of His adversary. We meet both in Genesis and in Revelation, at the beginning and at the end of the biblical story. Both the Tree of Life and the serpent are associated with the first man and the first women. At the Horite shrine of Heliopolis, the first couple Isis and Osiris were said to have emerged from the tree of life.

In the Gikuyu creation story we are told that at the beginning:

It was, our elders tell us, all dead except for the thunder, a violence that seemed to strangle life. It was this dark night whose depth you could not measure, not you nor I can conceive of its solid blackness, which would not let the sun pierce through it.

But in the darkness, at the foot of Mount Kerinyaga, a tree rose. At first it was a small tree and it grew up, finding a way even through the darkness. It wanted to reach the light and the sun. This tree had Life. It went up, sending forth the rich warmth of a blossoming tree - you know, a holy tree in the dark night of thunder and moaning. This was Mukuyu, God's tree.

Now you know that at the beginning of things there was only one man (Gikuyu) and one woman (Mumbi). It was under this Mukuyu that He first put them. And immediately the sun rose and the dark night melted away. The sun shone with a warmth that gave life and activity to all things.

The Tree of Life and the Tree of the Knowledge of Good and Evil

The Tree of Life is mentioned in Genesis 3:22 as distinct from the tree of the knowledge of good and evil. Both trees are mentioned in The Book of Enoch, a text sacred to Coptic Christians. In chapter 31 we read:

The tree of knowledge also was there, of which if any one eats, he becomes endowed with great wisdom. It was like a species of the tamarind tree, bearing fruit which resembled grapes extremely fine; and its fragrance extended to a considerable distance. I exclaimed, how beautiful is this tree, and how delightful is its appearance! Then holy Raphael, an

angel who was with me, answered and said, this is the tree
of knowledge, of which your ancient father and your aged
mother ate, who were before you; and who, obtaining
knowledge, their eyes being opened, and knowing themselves
to be naked, were expelled from the garden.

The tree of the knowledge of good and evil is another very ancient idea. The tree is often associated with the serpent. It may be that the coiled branches of certain trees that cause visions when consumed according to certain prescriptions looked like serpents.

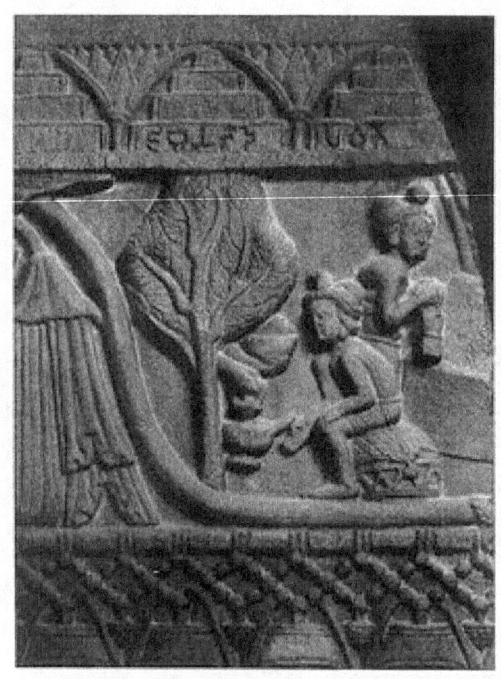

Left: Tree of Life with serpent on stone relief from India.

Healing for the Nations

The Book of Enoch also reports that at the great judgment God will give fruit from the Tree of Life to all whose names are in the Book of Life. This idea is also found in Revelation 2:7: "to him that overcometh will I give to eat of the tree of life, which is in the midst of the paradise of God."

In Matthew 13 Jesus describes the Kingdom of God as a tree that grows from a mustard seed. The branches shelter the birds who nest there. Likewise, the restoration of Paradise involves a Tree of Life which gives healing to those who are sheltered there.

If there is a tree in real time that serves as the basis for the Tree of Life, it might be the *Moringa oleifera* tree because it is the most nutritious source of plant-derived food found on the planet. Moringa is the Tamil-Dravidian name. The Hausa name for the tree is *Zogale*, meaning the *helper*. It is sometimes called the cabbage plant and is a stable in Afro-Arabian pharmacology.

For centuries, the natives of India, parts of Africa, Asia and South America have benefited from the Moringa's leaves, pods and flowers which are rich in nutrients important to humans and animals. The seeds are used to purify surface water and can produce a 90.00% to 99.99% bacterial reduction in previously untreated water.

Of course, none of this proves that the moringa tree and the Tree of Life are one and the same. I suppose it doesn't really matter, the fact is that the moringa tree is here and is a wonderful life and health giving tree whether it was the biblical tree of life or not!

Where does Moringa Grow Best?

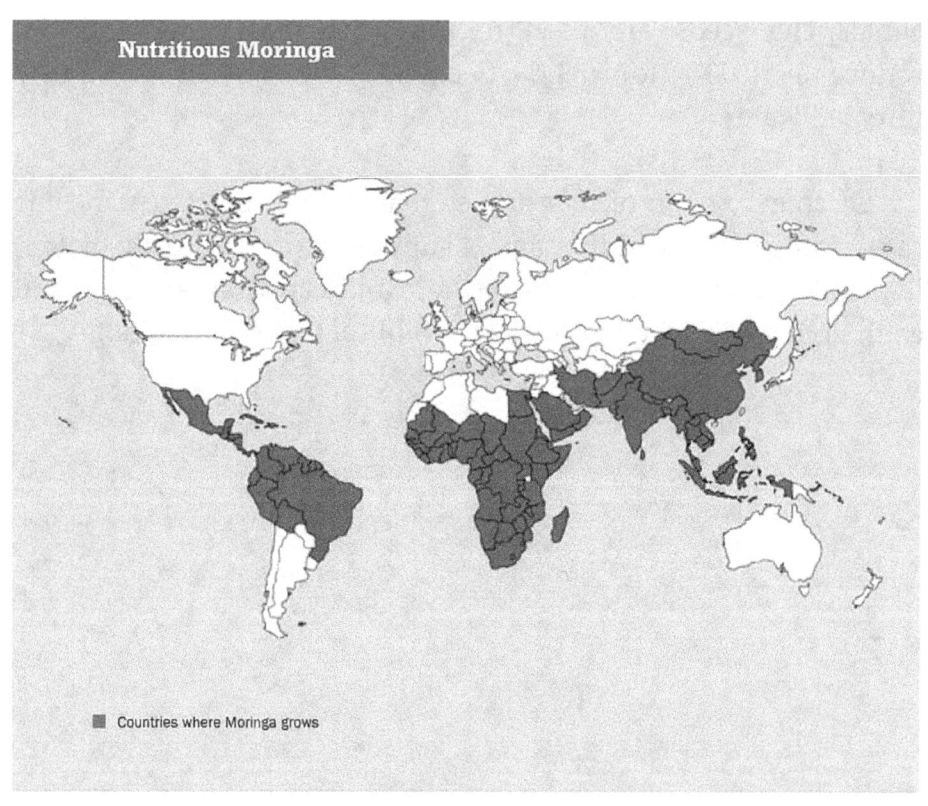

Nutritious Moringa

■ Countries where Moringa grows

The Moringa tree grows...

Right where it is needed most!

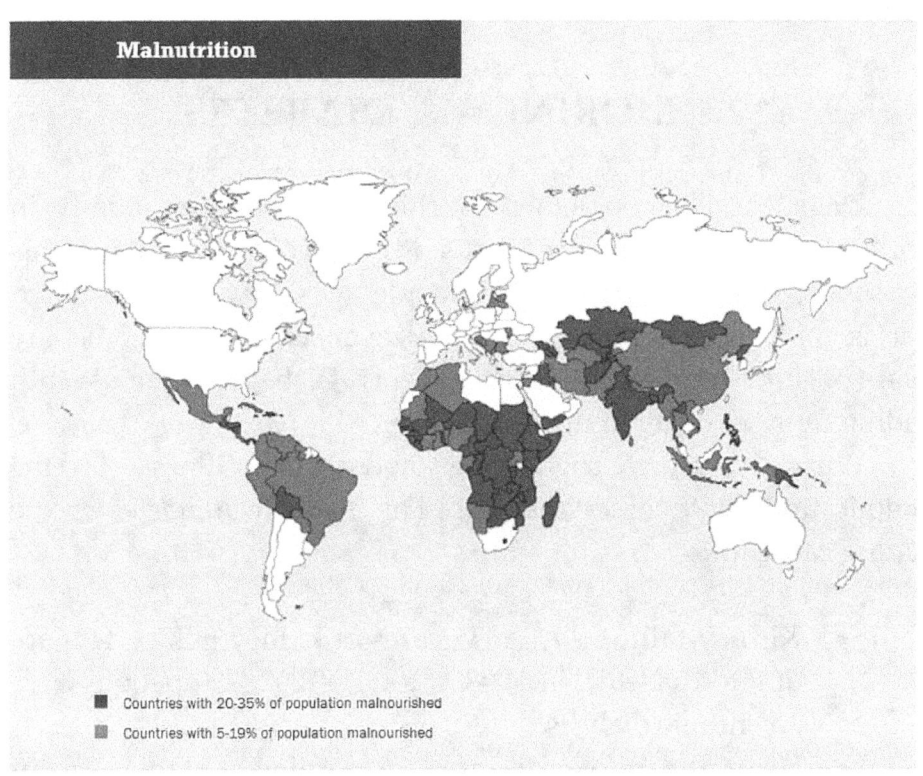

Malnutrition

- ■ Countries with 20-35% of population malnourished
- ▦ Countries with 5-19% of population malnourished

...precisely where people need it most.

12   MORINGA & DIABETES

Diabetes is an epidemic, touching almost every family in North America. Among residents in United States alone, this illness affects above 25.8 million people ages 20 years and older, that is 8.3% of the population. However very few people are aware on how moringa benefits diabetes. Diabetes is the seventh leading cause of death in the U.S.!

What is more frightening about this illness is the complications with other diseases. For example, diabetes is the leading cause for:

- **Kidney failure -** All new cases of kidney failure 44% are due to diabetes. In 2008, a total of 202, 290 people were on chronic dialysis.
- **Heart and Stroke disease -** According to statistics from 2004, 68% of diabetes-related deaths were by heart disease.
- **Lower limb amputations.**
- **New cases of blindness among the adult population**

Diabetes is a disease that is characterized by problems involving the hormone insulin. In healthy people, the pancreas releases insulin; insulin then works to help the body use and store the fat and sugar that is derived from the food that people eat. With diabetes, insulin can be compromised in a couple of different ways. In some cases, the pancreas doesn't produce any insulin at all. Other times, the body does not react in the right way to insulin - this is known as "insulin resistance." Finally, diabetes is sometimes characterized by a pancreas that produces an insufficient volume of insulin.

The two types of Diabetes -
It's important to understand that modern medical knowledge tells us that diabetes is a disease that has no cure. Once a person develops diabetes, they will suffer from the condition for the rest of their life. Although diabetes may be triggered by a variety of different phenomena involving the pancreas and insulin production - or lack thereof - it can also be divided into two distinct types.

<u>**Type 1 Diabetes**</u> - Type 1 diabetes typically first arises in people under the age of 20, although it can happen at any age. Insulin-producing cells - known as beta cells - in the pancreas are completely destroyed by the body's immune system. In turn, the pancreas can no longer produce any insulin and insulin injections must be administered.

Type 1 Diabetes

Healthy   Diabetic

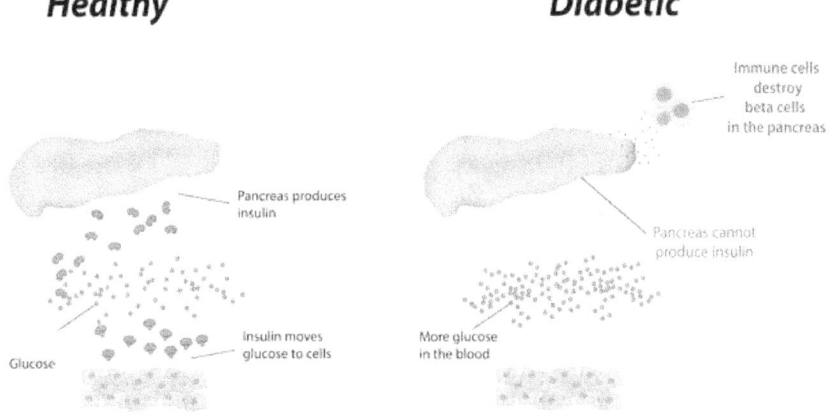

<u>Type 2 Diabetes</u> - With type 2 diabetes, a person's pancreas still produces insulin; the problem is that it either doesn't create enough insulin, or the person's body is resistant to the insulin that is produced. Type 2 diabetes commonly occurs in obese and overweight individuals - usually over the age of 40 - and is sometimes called "adult onset diabetes."

Type 2 Diabetes

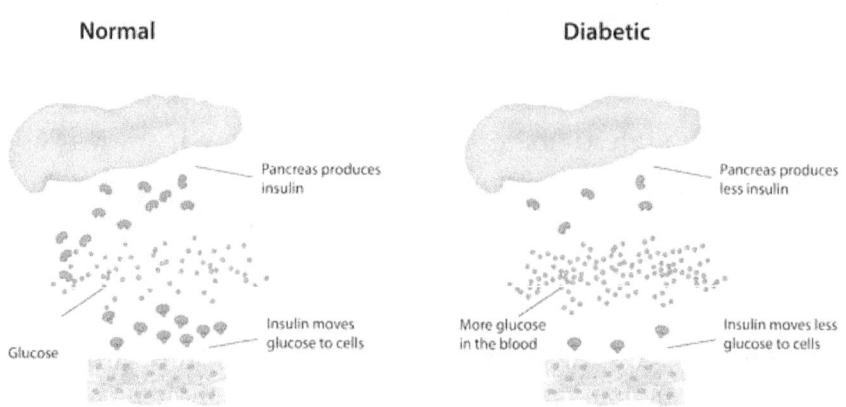

Managing Diabetes -

As noted above, modern medical science tells us that there is no cure for diabetes. However, there are several ways to manage the condition in order to keep insulin at the proper level. There are several different techniques and strategies for managing diabetes. Some of them include:

- carefully monitoring one's diet in order to keep blood sugar levels in check;
- using insulin injections as needed to maintain optimal levels in those whose bodies don't produce the hormone;

- keeping a close eye on blood sugar levels by using special kits that measure insulin and sugar in the blood; and

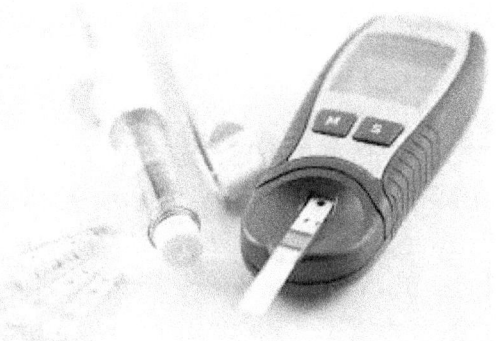

- following an exercise routine in order to keep blood pressure levels in check.

What Can Moringa do to Help –

As with any disease or condition, doctors and researchers are constantly seeking new ways to treat and manage diabetes. People are more concerned about using harsh, synthetic medications than ever before, which is what makes the promise of Moringa Oleifera all the more exciting. Moringa Oleifera is a tree that is originally native to India, but is now grown across the globe. As it happens, people in many developing countries - particular in Africa - have been using Moringa Oleifera to treat and manage the symptoms of diabetes for years with a good deal of success.

Simply put, diabetes is a metabolism disorder, were metabolism refers to the way our bodies use digested food for energy and growth. Most of what we consume is broken down into glucose, which makes its way into the bloodstream. However, to enable this smooth transition, the body needs insulin.

Insulin is a hormone produced in the pancreas. Blood sugar is regulated by insulin and is a main issue in diabetes. Many people who are living with diabetes have different ways of controlling their blood sugar levels. Some individuals use different medications to control diabetes, Other individuals might choose to modify their diets by lowering their carbohydrate and sugar intake. Most diabetics choose a combination of these two options.

The leaves of the Moringa oleifera tree contain a substantial amount of oleic acid. As with all of the other wonderful ingredients packed into Moringa leaves, this oleic acid is not processed or synthesized in any way, making it readily available for immediate absorption by the body. Oleic acid is an Omega-9 fatty acid that has been noted for its ability to, among other important things, help reduce the body's resistance to insulin and regulate levels of blood sugar. Oleic acid is the main ingredient in olive oil, which contains about 75% oleic acid and is the most widely available source of oleic acid.

In addition to containing high levels of oleic acid, Moringa oleifera leaves are full of other important nutrients that aid in combating diabetes. In fact, there is quite literally no plant species on planet Earth with a more densely packed profile of nutrients.

Diabetes retinopathy, or damage to the eyes from prolonged diabetes, occurs in approximately 40% of all Americans who are diagnosed with diabetes. This can lead to loss of vision and blindness over time. Moringa oleifera contains healthy amounts of vitamin A, much more than carrots offer in a serving for serving comparison, which has been shown to build the strength of the cornea, stop eye inflammation, and decrease the risk of macular degeneration.

Vitamin C is important for proper production and regulation of insulin. A deficiency in vitamin C has been shown to adversely affect the ability of the pancreas to secrete insulin, which contributes to higher levels of blood sugar. Moringa contains high levels of vitamin C, more per serving than orange juice, which helps the pancreas secrete insulin at normal levels.

Other vitamins and minerals have also been shown to help in the production and regulation of insulin, both in the pancreas and elsewhere around the body. For example, vitamin E has been shown in several studies to decrease the risk of developing diabetes. Moringa has 3 times more Vitamin E than is found in almonds. A powerful antioxidant, vitamin E makes it easier for the body to transport and manage insulin by improving the integrity of cell membranes. Research

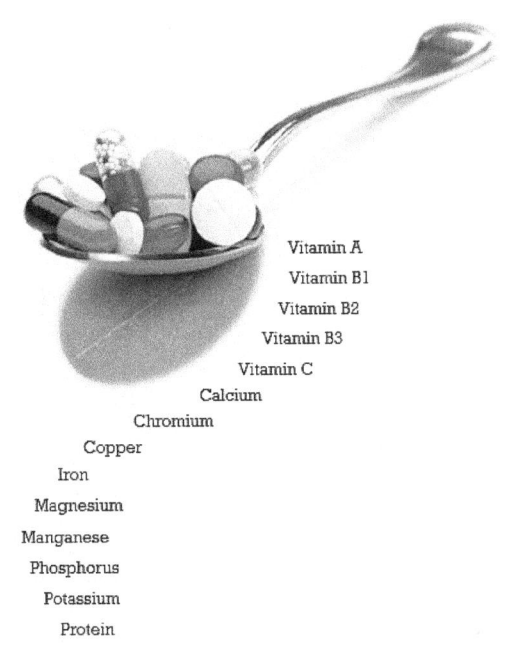

Vitamin A
Vitamin B1
Vitamin B2
Vitamin B3
Vitamin C
Calcium
Chromium
Copper
Iron
Magnesium
Manganese
Phosphorus
Potassium
Protein
Zinc

studies have found the importance of having an intake of 400 IU of Vitamin E daily, thereby lowering cardiovascular risk by as much as 50%. Rich with vitamin E, and more than 40 other powerful antioxidants, Moringa can help to improve your body's management and regulation of blood sugar on a cellular level and provide you with a full spectrum of nutrients to balance the effects of diabetes.

- Vitamin B 12 is also found in Moringa leaves, which is used successfully to treat the "neuropatia diabetic".
- Lack of Vitamin D contributes the risk in children to developing Type One Diabetes. New studies have shown that kids living above the latitude 40 have a higher risk in developing juvenile diabetes (Type One). Vitamin D protects

the insulin cell producers, when the level of vitamin D is low, the body will become insulin dependent for life.

- Moringa has 4 times more Calcium than milk and 3 times more Potassium than Bananas.

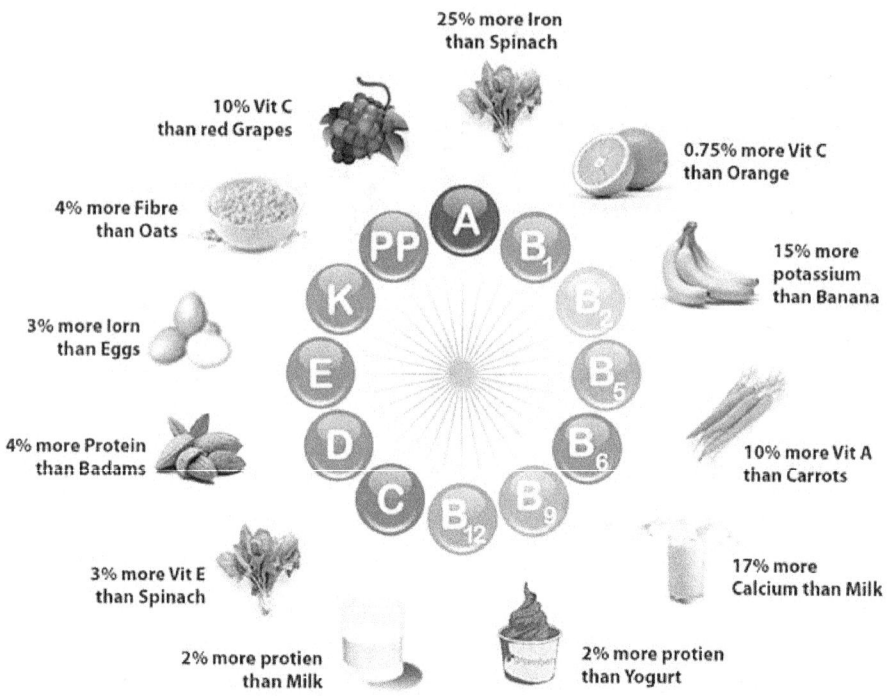

In Asia and Africa, the Moringa leaf is hailed as a cure-all. Although it is most commonly used to treat malnutrition in developing countries, many doctors recognise that the Moringa leaf can help over 300 diseases, including diabetes. Despite these claims, people in the Western Hemisphere know little about this natural supplement's possible benefits.

The Moringa leaf is a nutrient powerhouse because it possesses large quantities of vitamins A, C, calcium, iron, and protein. I already mentioned that due in large part to its abundance of vitamin A, Moringa may prevent diabetic retinopathy. This is significant because 28.5% of people over 40 with diabetes have developed diabetic retinopathy between 2005 and 2008. Moringa is also rich in vitamin C. Combined with insulin, vitamin C can halt blood vessel damage in people with Type 1 diabetes, decreasing their risk for chest pain, heart attack, and stroke.

Some users credit the Moringa herb for reducing tumor size and blood pressure. The supplement can also boost your immune system. For people with diabetes, these benefits could be significant due to their increased risk for heart disease and cancer. For people with insulin resistance, dangerously high levels of blood glucose could cause excessive amounts of inflammation, resulting in limited blood flow. This lack of blood flow can lead to a heart attack or stroke. Weight management is another potential pro in taking Moringa leaf because of the amount of protein it possesses -- foods high in protein can reduce cravings in between meals.

VITAMINS

Vitamin A (α-carotene and β-carotene), B1, B2, B3, B5, B6, C, E, K, Folic Acid

MINERALS

Calcium, Chloride, Chromium, Copper, Flourine, Iron, Maganese, Magnesium, Molybendum, Phosphorus, Potassium, Sodium, Selenium, Sulfur, Zinc

OTHER NUTRIENTS

Chlorophyll, Carotenoids, Cytokins, Flavonoids, Omega 3 - 6 - 9 Oils, Plant Sterols, Polyphenols, Lutein, Xanthins, Rutin and many more.

18 AMINO ACIDS

Isoleucine, Leucine, Lysine, Methionine, Phenylalanine, Threonine, Tryptophan, Valine, Alanine, Arginine, Aspartic Acid, Cystine, Glycine Glutamine, , Histidine, Proline, Serine, Tyrosine

46 ANTI-OXIDANTS

Alanine, Beta-sitosterol, Caffeoylquinic Acid, Campesterol, Carotenoids, Chlorophyll, Delta-5-Avenasterol, Delta-7-Avenasterol, Glutathione, Indole Acetic Acid, Indoleacetonitrile, Kaempferal, Lutein, Methionine, Myristic-Acid, Palmitic-Acid, Prolamine, Proline, Quercetin, Rutin, Selenium, Threonine, Tryptophan, Xanthins, Xanthophyll, Zeatin, Zeaxanthin and more.

36 ANTI-INFLAMMATORY COMPOUNDS

Moringa leaves can be eaten raw, cooked, or made into powder. While some people claim that raw Moringa leaves taste like radishes, cooked Moringa is said to be more similar to spinach. Using Moringa powder in your tea can also provide you with a quick and natural boost of energy.

Lots of information has been written about Moringa and diabetes; however, there is not enough scientific research to substantiate its claim as a diabetes cure. But what is certain is that it could provide people with diabetes additional assistance by reducing their likelihood of developing other illnesses. For these reasons and more, it is important to add Moringa to your diet. But remember, it is also very important to consult your doctor before incorporating Moringa leaf into your diet to treat diabetes.

Why does Moringa Oleifera hold so much promise for those who suffer from diabetes?

Primarily because of its many amazing, natural benefits, Moringa Oleifera has been shown to naturally boost the immune system, which usually becomes compromised in those who suffer from type 1 and type 2 diabetes. Moringa Oleifera has also been shown to possess many key anti-inflammatory benefits; diabetes often causes circulatory problems which can be managed through anti-inflammatory supplements. There are no negative side effects associated with Moringa Oleifera use, meaning that it is a safe, natural way for people to manage their blood sugar and care for their diabetes symptoms. It's just one more option for the many people who have to cope with this serious condition.

13 MORINGA & HEART HEALTH

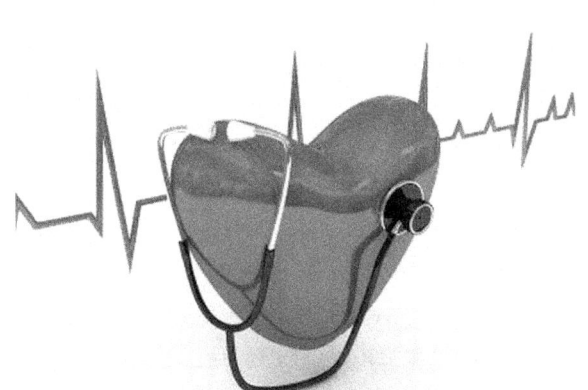

Cardiovascular disease is a major health issue worldwide and predicted by 2020 to be the most common threat to human life, the ultimate cause of death being myocardial infarction (heart attack). It is thus important to take precautions to protect the heart through a healthy diet and lifestyle. With recent interest in exploring the cardioprotective potential of natural products, numerous studies have been conducted that determine overall effectiveness of *Moringa Oleifera* in maintaining a healthy heart through its provision of vitamins, minerals and Phytonutrient that can protect the heart and lower blood pressure.

Moringa is chock full of antioxidants which are substances that remove the toxic byproducts of chemical reactions in our bodies. That's why you hear so much about antioxidants - they are responsible for clearing out highly reactive chemicals that circulate in the body, making sure they don't cause DNA, cell, or tissue damage. It is this damage that is believed to cause heart disease, cancer and premature aging. The antioxidant and free radical scavenging properties of moringa give way to its cardioprotective capabilities. Previous studies that simulate human heart disease in rat models have found that the damages to the heart that ultimately lead to a heart attack involve the formation of oxygen-free radicals. Free radicals weaken the protective membranes in the body and thus can weaken the heart to the point of a myocardial infarction. However, in rats pretreated with *Moringa Oleifera* leaf extract, the presence of free radicals was significantly reduced, proving the anti-oxidative and protective property of moringa (Panda et al. 2012).

It's not just the antioxidants we need that moringa offers, there are loads of vitamins too. Of all the essential nutrients that our bodies need on a regular basis, vitamins are perhaps the most researched and well-known. Ever since we were children, we were told of the importance of taking our vitamins. These nutrients help our body perform hundreds of different functions and without we simply cannot survive. Vitamins for cardiac health are specific vitamins which contribute to overall heart health and function, while helping prevent heart disease and other cardiovascular issues.

The most important group of vitamins specifically for heart health is the B Vitamin Family. These vitamins serve specific functions that can significantly reduce your risk of developing heart disease. The B Vitamins present in Moringa, specifically folic acid (Vitamin B9), Vitamin B6 and Vitamin B12 are all responsible for helping the body remove homocysteine from the blood. High levels of homocysteine can cause artery damage. Meat is a

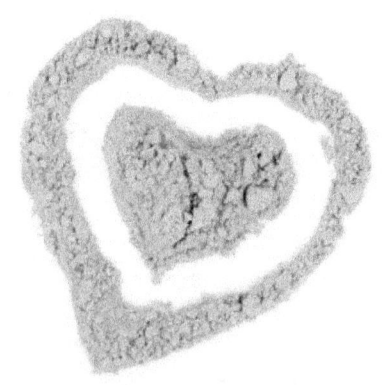

good source of B vitamins, which is why vegetarians have an increased risk of dangerous homocysteine levels. It is especially important that they supplement these important vitamins for cardiac health. Vitamin B3 in Moringa, known more commonly as niacin, may also reduce cholesterol in high concentrations, although further testing is needed to prove this conclusively. As far as other heart vitamins are concerned, the Vitamin E and Vitamin C in Moringa work in conjunction with each other to prevent heart disease and other ailments through their antioxidant abilities.

As I mentioned above, another vitamin for cardiac health is folic acid (also a member of the B family of vitamins – vitamin B9) which is known to reduce the risk of coronary heart disease and stroke, according to a detailed analysis of more than three dozen scientific studies. Great news – Moringa has tons of folic acid to offer! These nutrients work by quenching homocysteine, an amino acid in the blood that attacks blood vessel walls and promotes cardiovascular disease. Homocysteine (pronounced ho'-mo-sis'-teen) has emerged after 25 years of research as the "new cholesterol," and researchers estimate that it is a major risk factor in 10 to 40 percent of heart attacks and strokes in the United States. Under normal circumstances, this amino acid is a short-lived byproduct of methionine metabolism, but a diet short on B vitamins prevents its breakdown.

The latest study, published in the Journal of the American Medical Association, analyzed 38 previous studies on homocysteine, folic acid, and cardiovascular diseases. Researcher Shirley A. A. Beresford, PhD, of the University of Washington, confirmed that high blood levels of homocysteine were clearly associated with cardiovascular diseases and that folic acid lowered levels of the amino acid. Other studies have reported that vitamins for cardiac health also include B6, B12, and choline also lower homocysteine levels. High blood levels of homocysteine, also known as hyperhomocysteinemia, pose a risk of cardiovascular disease independent of other risk factors, such as cholesterol, triglyceride, smoking, and so forth. Beresford estimated that up to 50,000 coronary heart disease deaths could be prevented every year by increasing folic acid intake; by eating more fruit and vegetables, fortifying foods with the vitamin, and including moringa in the diet.

Moringa is well documented as being great at reducing inflammation in the human body – but what does that really mean?

A great question! One of moringa's key benefits is its ability to reduce inflammation. This anti-inflammatory action is due to the fact that it is rich in powerful anti-inflammatory compounds like isothiocyanates, flavonoids, and phenolic acids.

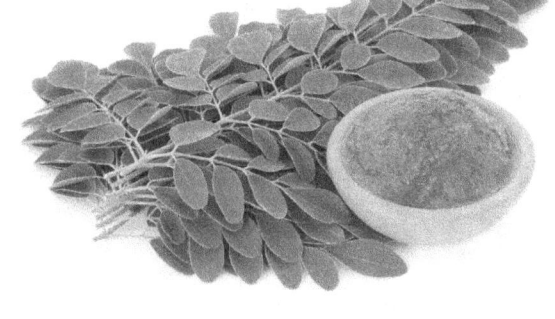

Its potent anti-inflammatory action is the reason why moringa is traditionally used to treat stomach ulcers. The sweet tasting moringa oil, derived from pressing the leaves, pods and seeds (sometimes called Ben oil) has also been shown to protect the liver from chronic inflammation.

In 2012, the discovery that inflammation in artery walls is the **true cause** of heart disease led to many mainstream experts, like world-renowned heart surgeon Dr. Dwight Lundell, speaking out against the current measures used to prevent heart disease: such as prescribing side effect-ridden statin drugs to everyone that is over the age of 40 – even to those with no heart disease risk factors.

The fact is, without inflammation present in the body, there is no way that cholesterol would accumulate in artery walls, causing heart disease and strokes. Without inflammation, cholesterol can move freely throughout the body as nature intended. It is inflammation that causes cholesterol to become trapped. Moringa helps to reduce inflammation.

Despite what we've been told for years, cholesterol is not the villain it is made out to be and instead of lowering this essential compound in our bodies to ridiculously low levels, what we should be doing is fighting inflammation (without drugs) and maintaining a healthy balance between HDL and LDL cholesterol levels – both of these serve essential functions in our bodies.

In both instances, incorporating moringa leaf, powder, or oil, into our diets can benefit your heart health tremendously. Apart from its potent anti-inflammatory properties, moringa has also been found to help maintain healthy cholesterol levels. In fact, in Thai traditional medicine moringa is used as a cardio-tonic. Recent studies have demonstrated its benefits for those suffering with hereditary hypocholesterolaemia – extremely high cholesterol levels that can pose other health risks like the calcification of arteries.

In these studies, consuming moringa outperformed one of the most prescribed statin drugs, simvastatin, by bringing high cholesterol levels back to healthy levels and reducing atherosclerotic plaque formation (responsible for the calcification of arteries) by 50 and 86 per cent, respectively.

If you live in the UK or the US, getting your hands on a moringa tree can be tricky, and growing one in your backyard garden may not be a feasible option either, I understand that, however, if you have access to a moringa tree, you can use the fresh leaves, similar in flavor to radish, in your meals. Toss them like a salad, blend them into smoothies, or steam them like spinach.

Another option is to use Moringa powder (found at specialist alternative health food stores), either in supplement form or added to smoothies, soups, and other foods for extra nutrition. Some people find that Moringa powder has a distinctive "green" flavor, so you may want to start out slowly when adding it to your meals.

Finally, organic, cold-pressed moringa oil (or Ben Oil), can also be used in salad dressings and topically to treat antifungal problems and arthritis, it is also an excellent skin moisturizer. It is true that Moringa oil is expensive – about 15 times more than olive oil – but considering the heart health benefits you'll get from taking moringa it seems like a small price to pay.

Several studies have been conducted with rodents to determine the effect of Moringa on heart health. When administered to lab rats at a dose of 200 mg/kg/day for one month, Moringa was shown to significantly protect the heart, improve its function, and prevent the accumulation of lipid peroxides that cause cell damage. Thus, further clinical studies are warranted to support the therapeutic use of Moringa in ischemic heart disease in humans (Nandave et al. 2009). These studies are planned for the near future.

Maintaining a healthy heart requires a protective diet. These studies have proven Moringa can contribute to the protection of the heart and is an excellent way to integrate high-quality nutrition and valuable antioxidants into a heart-healthy diet.

More and more, our concern for heart health encompasses many aspects of our lives. Because our circulatory system connects every organ, tissue and cell in our bodies, many factors play a role in keeping hearts healthy and beating happily. These factors include: good nutrition for a properly functioning heart and healthy blood, physical activity to supply oxygen to blood, smart lifestyle choices and stress management.

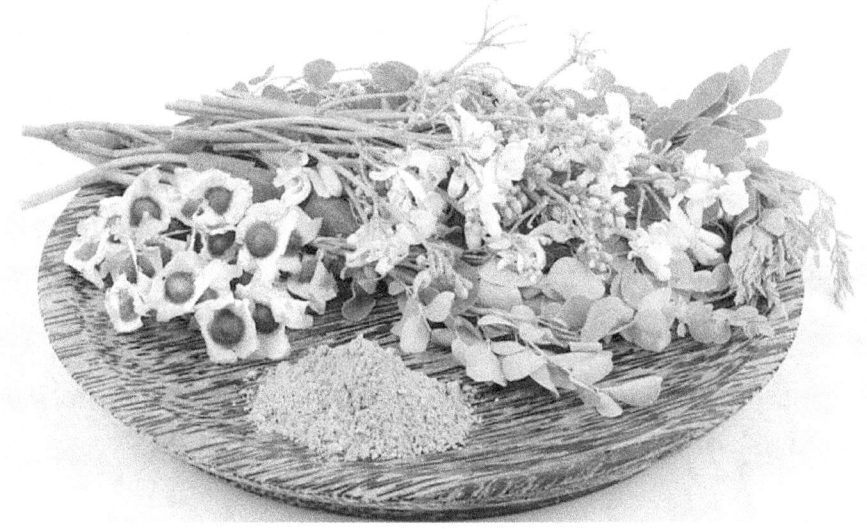

Excellent nutrition is essential to good heart health. Our hearts work hard every day to pump blood throughout our bodies so we have to do our part in helping our hearts along. Namely, we have to fuel our hearts with only the best nutrients to keep it going for many years to come. Many studies have shown that the best nutrients for our heart health are found in abundance in Moringa and include:

- **Omega-3 Fatty Acids -** that supply EPA and DHA, which can prevent blood clots, keep blood pressure in check, reduce inflammation and manage cholesterol levels. The top food choice for omega-3 fatty acids is fish, such as salmon or tuna.
- **B Vitamins -** aid in keeping red blood cells and nerves healthy. It may also lower homocysteine, a non-protein amino acid in the blood that is linked to heart attacks, blood clots and

strokes. B Vitamins are commonly found in bran, pistachios and hazelnuts, certain types of seeds, fish and spices, including garlic.

- **Magnesium** - helps hearts beat regularly and is often used to treat heart arrhythmia. Magnesium, found in walnuts, is also vital to all of our other organs as well.
- **Fiber** - especially from whole grains, is a great asset for cardiovascular health and has been associated with lowering the risk of heart disease. Fiber can also reduce harmful LDL cholesterol levels. Breads, rice, wheat and grain products are all excellent sources of fiber. Fiber also helps the body feel satiated, which may help to reduce one's overall caloric intake.
- **Quercetin** - is an anti-oxidant that helps prevent blood from clotting. It is naturally found in apples and can help to lower the risk of heart disease.

It's important to eat lean proteins, lots of fruits and vegetables and whole grains to reap the benefits for your heart, but Moringa can ensure you are on a heart-healthy path each and every day.

The Clinical Council on Cardiology says that after a heart-healthy diet, daily exercise is a key factor in maintaining heart health. Exercise increases the heart rate and gets oxygen flowing through the blood, invigorating the body. Studies have also proven that high intensity exercise can reduce LDL cholesterol. Additionally, exercise helps with weight management and maintaining a healthy body mass index, a strong indicator for avoiding cardiovascular disease. Moringa also aids in both exercise and weight management by providing the body with the energy it needs for physical activity, helping to repair broken down muscle tissues, and supplying excellent nutrition to help you feel satiated while revving up your metabolism.

Lastly, lifestyle choices and stress can impact heart health. Smoking is a major cause of heart disease-related heart attacks and strokes. Stress creates a chemical reaction in the body that can increase blood pressure and have a host of other negative physical and emotional consequences. When stress takes hold of our lives, we are more likely to overeat or make poor nutritional choices and be depressed and lethargic. Making positive lifestyle choices that improve our heart health, like not smoking and managing stress, can go a long way in keeping the beats healthy and happy.

A growing body of scientific research indicates that what we eat and drink can protect our body against a slew of health afflictions. Studies show that nearly 70% of heart disease cases are preventable when we make the right food choices. One "right" food choice is the Moringa Oleifera.

Nutritionists as well as health and fitness experts the world over are now touting the Moringa tree as being the perfect food for our body.

"What's good for your heart is good for your brain and good for you in general," says Arthur Agatston, MD, a renowned cardiologist and founder of the South Beach Diet.

Moringa Benefits

Discovered in the southern foothills of the Himalayas in northwestern India, the Moringa Oleifera tree is gaining worldwide acclaim for its remarkable nutritional and medicinal benefits. In fact, the leaves of the Moringa tree have no equal in the plant kingdom. It is recognized by most experts as the most nutritious food in the world, with most of its benefits stored in the small green leaves of this unpretentious plant.

Known in many cultures as the "Tree of Life," it contains more than 90 nutrients, including 46 powerful antioxidants and 18 amino acids. In fact, practically every part of the plant contains important minerals and are a good source of protein, vitamins, beta-carotene, flavonoids, and various phenolics.

In gram for gram comparisons to common fruits and vegetables, Moringa leaves contain:
- 7 times the vitamin C in oranges
- 4 times the calcium in milk and twice the protein
- 4 times the vitamin A in carrots
- 3 times the iron found in almonds
- And 3 times the potassium in bananas

We have already discussed the importance of antioxidants in our diets. Because of the significant volume and variety of antioxidants, Moringa is excellent for heart health. Antioxidants help keep your blood vessels strong and elastic. An easy way to tell if they're doing their job is to measure the amount of homocysteine in your blood. Normal levels of it are fairly harmless. But if your body doesn't get enough antioxidants or your antioxidant systems are overwhelmed, homocysteine levels rise.

Too much homocysteine in your blood can deteriorate your artery walls leading to plaque buildup and inflammation. It can also make it difficult for your blood vessels to dilate, thus blocking blood flow to the heart. One way to clean out excess homocysteine is with antioxidants and B vitamins – and as I told you above, Moringa has both.

Dr. Levette Truette, writing for the University of Florida News, says, "Almost all diseases can be prevented or destroyed if given enough antioxidants. In fact, Moringa has every single essential nutrient required for humans . . . and also contains every essential and non-essential amino acid that humans require."

According to an August 2004 article in the *Journal of the American Medical Association*, antioxidants, like vitamin E for instance, one of many antioxidants in Moringa leaves, slows the progression of atherosclerosis, or hardening of the arteries. Also, one of the amino acids contained in Moringa is a key factor in preventing cardiovascular disease.

MORINGA TRUMPS SUPERFOOD RIVALS IN **ORAC** TESTS

	ORAC Value (µ mole TE/100g)
• Moringa oleifera	157,600
• Matcha tea	134,800
• Turmeric, ground	127,068
• Acai, fruit	102,700
• Dark chocolate	20,800
• Garlic, raw	5,700
• Red wine	3,600
• Green tea	1,240

Oxygen Radical Absorbance Capacity (or ORAC value score) is a measurement of antioxidants in foods and supplements.

One of the most common cardiovascular diseases is high blood pressure or what's also referred to as *hypertension*. To say it's "common" is fairly accurate because more people see their doctor for high blood pressure than for any other reason. High blood pressure is dangerous because it makes the heart work harder to pump blood to the body. As the pressure builds inside our arteries, veins, and capillaries, our heart becomes even more overworked. Over time, our heart grows larger in an effort to compensate for the extra workload and eventually becomes weaker.

High blood pressure also damages the endothelium, the thin lining inside our artery walls, hurting the body's ability to produce nitric oxide (NO). NO is necessary to lower blood pressure because it relaxes the blood vessels and increases blood flow.

A key amino acid found in Moringa is L-Arginine. It is a precursor for the production of NO. When the body produces healthy levels of NO, you remain heart healthy. With its supply of L-Arginine, Moringa leaves help the body in its vital production of NO. Meanwhile, the antioxidants contained in the leaves help protect and stabilize the nitric oxide, thereby further enhancing the levels of nitric oxide.

Moringa Supplements Abound as Awareness Increases

Since early 2012, the popularity of Moringa in the U.S. exploded when Dr. Oz, a popular medical doctor began promoting Moringa nutritional supplements on his daytime TV program as an "energy blaster" and a great way to "jump start your day." Because of this plant's remarkable antioxidant, anti-inflammatory, anti-aging and energy-enhancing qualities, this physician recommends taking Moringa Oleifera capsules daily.

With more people clamoring for Moringa to take advantage of its staggering array of nutritional and medicinal benefits, many nutritional supplement companies have jumped on the bandwagon to meet the rapidly growing demand. Moringa supplements now proliferate across the U.S. market.

There's a bit of a problem with this picture, however.

Not all Moringa supplements are made from FRESH leaves . . . nor do they come from trees grown in the rich Himalayan soil of northwestern India. Scientific analysis shows that only trees from this region contain the **highest** nutritional potency. And not are all Moringa supplements are made to the highest standards . . . nor provide the highest level of effectiveness possible.

This leaves many consumers asking:

"How to choose a Moringa supplement?"

The answer is simple (sort of). Select the supplement whose Moringa leaves are picked fresh and whole from trees grown in the Himalayan foothills . . . washed and sorted within hours to preserve ALL their nutrients, then immediately dehydrated and steam treated for purity before being milled into powder and encapsulated. A supplement that uses no extracts, no fillers, or "other ingredients," but which delivers only the freshest, most nutrient rich Moringa available in the market today. This sounds easier than it turns out to be, my advice is to find a main-stream supplement supplier with a good reputation and years of honest business behind it.

However you choose to include Moringa into your diet my best advice is to just do it! As I always caution...

I Am Not A Doctor

The information presented here is accurate to the best of my knowledge.

I am not a doctor therefore this information is not intended to diagnose, treat, cure or prevent any disease because only doctors can do that.

Please do your own research!

14   Moringa & Alzheimer's

Dementia, Alzheimer's disease, and memory loss, these are all Neurodegenerative diseases and all are a part of the ageing process and will eventually touch all of us in some way, right? No, No, NO!

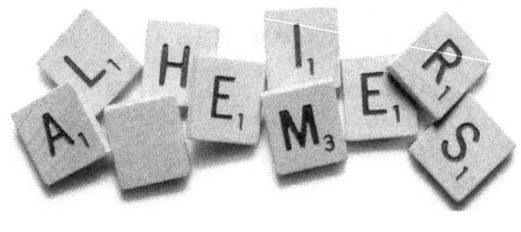 While it may seem to be a normal part of getting older, memory loss and other neurodegenerative diseases need not be something you worry about. We do not have all of the answers yet but what we have learned so far tells us that we can fight these debilitating conditions years before they set their sights on us. And we can do it from the inside out by choosing what foods we eat.

Adding Moringa to your diet will help you fight many issues with brain function and memory long before the problems begin to affect your life. Our ability to employ preventive methods against Neurodegenerative diseases is incredibly important due, not only, to the rapid growth of these diseases in the modern world, but also due to humanity living longer, the rising costs of medical care, and the understanding that dementia need not be a 'normal' part of the

PROJECTED RISE IN ALZHEIMER'S CASES BY 2025

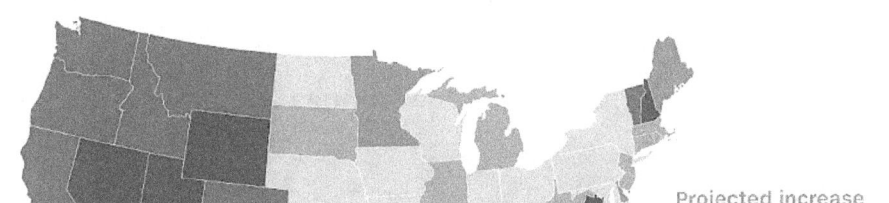

Projected increase

14.3% - 21.6%
21.7% - 26.4%
26.5% - 34.8%
34.9% - 44.1%
44.2% - 71.9%

SOURCE: Alzheimer's Association

ageing process. Not only that, but having the option that we can eat foods specifically to combat these conditions gives us some amount of control over our future health. This is especially welcome since we live in a time when modern medical science offers therapeutic treatments for dementia that are actually extremely limited.

Modern scientific research has shown us that oxidative stress plays a big part in brain health. In fact, we now know that it not only plays a role but it plays a crucial role in our mental and cognitive abilities. The effects of many herbs were studied with respect to age-related dementia and the antioxidant activity they offered. The neuro enhancing activities of Moringa Oleifera have proven to be more significant, with respect to improving spatial memory, than nearly any other plants studied.

Neuro protection with Moringa Oleifera leaf extract in animal models is very promising. Science has now learned that Moringa leaf extract is an important cognitive enhancer and neuroprotectant. This ability of Moringa may well be due, at least partly, to the decreased oxidative stress and enhanced cholinergic function that results from consuming Moringa. However, further studies on the active ingredients in Moringa leaf powder are yet to be conducted.

Dementia is a condition in which a serious loss of global cognitive ability happens. This often includes memory, attention, and language impairments. In some people, it also affects problem solving ability that continues to increase as the person ages. Recent findings 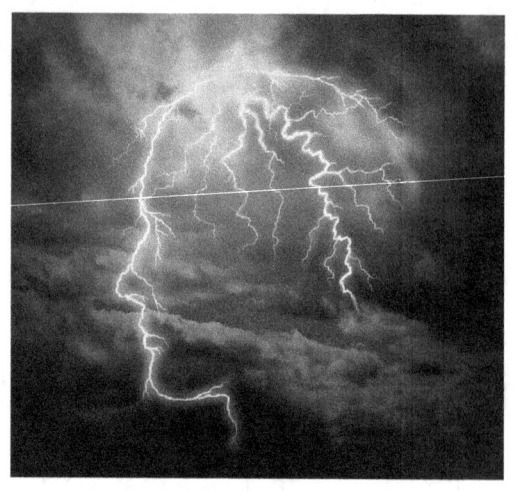 have shown that the age-related cognitive dysfunction occurs as a result of oxidative stress. It has been responsible for the increase of stress hormones in the brain.

While many believe that studying the effects, on the brain, of various new drugs, is the right approach to dementia treatment, not all agree. Researchers that disagree point out that most drugs still induce adverse side-effects. This disadvantage consequently motivates their research efforts to look for other, novel, more natural, protective agents against dementia. Basically, that means looking to herbal medicine. The problem here is that many in the scientific community look at traditional herbal medicine as tantamount to witchcraft. That is a real shame because herbal medicine has long been used to treat numerous ailments, and the general population, when threatened with the side effects of so many modern drugs, often prefers natural produces and extracts. These herbal products often offer more advantages than synthetic drugs. More and more lines of evidence have demonstrated, beyond doubt, that eating Phytonutrient-rich foods containing antioxidant-dense qualities enhance cognitive performance in elderly subjects. This is conclusively proven, it is not theory, speculation, or wishful thinking.

Simply put, we now know, beyond a shadow of a doubt, that eating good quality, fresh, nutrient rich foods, leads to better health both now and into the future.

Moringa has compounds such as tannins, phenolics, alkaloids, saponins and steroids, which all fight against oxidative stress. The Moringa Oleifera plant is highly regarded by dieticians and medical researchers and practitioners due to its superior nutritional content and numerous medical applications. The antioxidant properties of the moringa plant have been well established by previous medical studies and are believed to provide protection against the effects of oxidative stress and free radicals that can cause aging and other negative health effects. Recent studies suggest that moringa leaves can also provide protection against the symptoms of Alzheimer's disease and may even delay its onset.

Alzheimer's disease is believed to have a genetic component but can strike even those with no family history of the disease. Most cases of Alzheimer's occur in individuals over 65 years of age, but the disease can strike much earlier in cases of 'early-onset' Alzheimer's disease. As in other types of dementia, the patient experiences confusion, loss of normal brain function, unpredictable or aggressive tendencies and a gradual deterioration of the mental capacities. This degeneration of the nervous system eventually leads to death. While the exact causes of Alzheimer's disease are

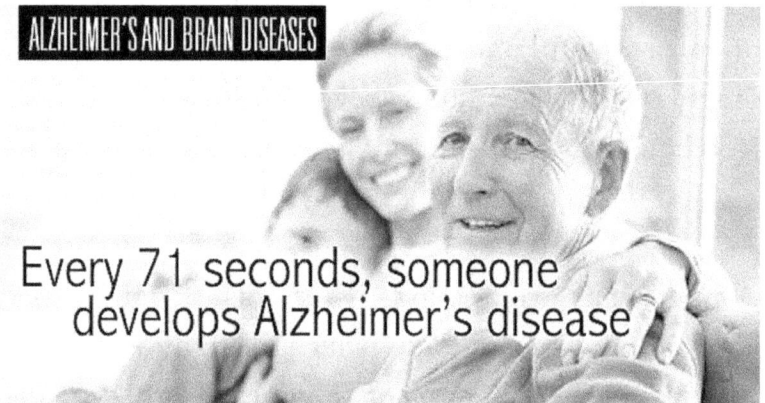

ALZHEIMER'S AND BRAIN DISEASES

Every 71 seconds, someone develops Alzheimer's disease

not well understood, research studies seem to indicate that the disease is related to the build-up of fibrous protein compounds within the brain known as amyloids. These amyloids present within the brain as plaques or neurofibrillary tangles and are thought to disrupt the normal functioning of neural impulses within the brain.

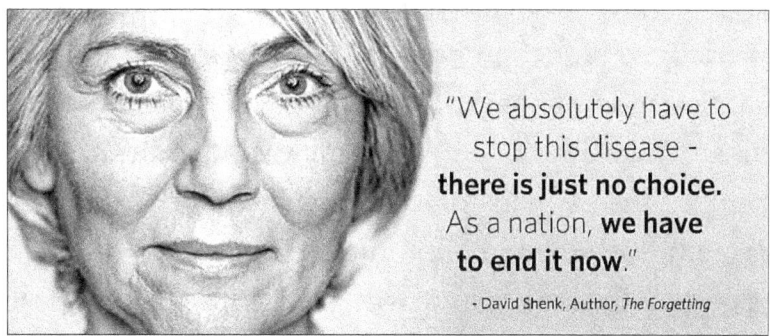

"We absolutely have to stop this disease - **there is just no choice.** As a nation, **we have to end it now**."

- David Shenk, Author, *The Forgetting*

Because there is no known cure for Alzheimer's disease, most treatments focus on delaying the progress of the disease and alleviating symptoms. Natural treatments including Moringa and medical marijuana have produced impressive results in preventing continued degeneration. Other treatments focus on improving the emotional state of the patient and controlling any aggressive or violent tendencies that may occur due to the deteriorating mental condition. Although the precise causes of Alzheimer's disease are not yet known, a number of correlating factors have been identified that may be responsible for triggering or worsening Alzheimer's in some patients. These factors include the age and gender of the patient, the use of cigarettes and alcohol, genetic factors, congenital conditions including Down's syndrome and multiple sclerosis, and the overall level of fat intake by the patient. Most of these factors are not directly under the control of the individual at risk for the disease.

Lifestyle changes are often recommended in order to help

delay or prevent the onset of Alzheimer's disease. These include smoking cessation strategies, reduction of alcohol consumption and, especially, a reduction in fat intake. It is in the latter area that Moringa has been shown to be most useful in delaying or preventing Alzheimer's in vulnerable individuals. A study published in the Annals of Neurosciences in 2005 showed a significant improvement in brain function in rats whose diets were supplemented by moringa leaves prior to their exposure to colchicine, a substance that mimics the action of Alzheimer's in the brain. Despite the presence of this substance, rats retained much of their cognitive abilities and navigated a previously-completed maze far more accurately and quickly than the control group. These results were attributed to the antioxidant properties of moringa leaves, which served to scavenge free radicals from the system and to protect neural function.

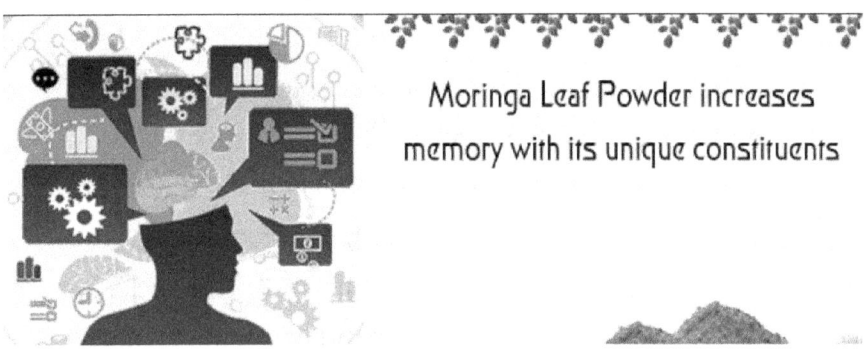

Moringa Leaf Powder increases memory with its unique constituents

Moringa leaves appear to delay or mitigate the effects of Alzheimer's disease in laboratory rats due to the supplement's antioxidant effects. The research indicates that moringa supplements may lessen the impact of Alzheimer's in individuals already suffering from the disease and may delay or prevent its onset in those who are at risk of developing this devastating illness. By incorporating moringa leaf supplements into daily dietary plans, it is likely that most individuals can improve their chances of avoiding the worst effects of Alzheimer's disease and other Neurodegenerative diseases for themselves and their families.

Conclusion – In My Opinion

This is the conclusion of my book. The "rules" of proper book layout and publishing demand that in the conclusion I sum up all of the preceding chapters and answer any questions that may still remain in the minds of my readers.

Frankly I do not want to do that.
So, since I have never much been one for following all the "rules," I think I'll approach this chapter the way I want.

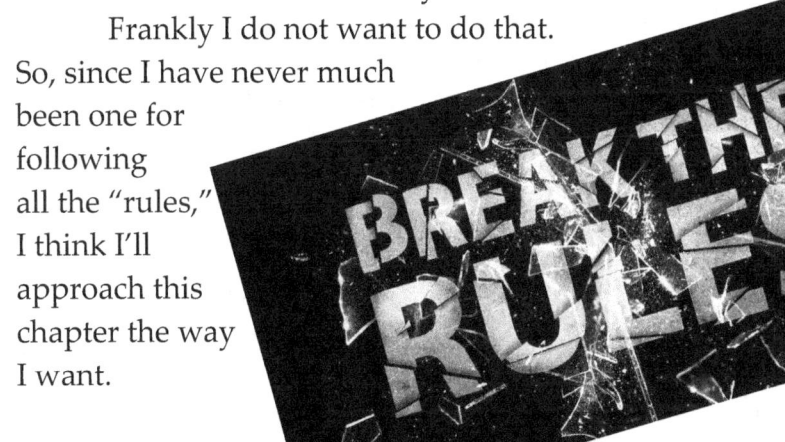

You see, I
absolutely do not
want to answer all   of your questions with this book. In
fact, I think that all of those so called, "all you need to know" books
are ridiculous!

What I want to achieve with this work, what hope I have achieved is that I provided you with enough solid, scientific information that you are encouraged to start asking even more questions about the amazing Miracle Tree. I hope you do some research of your own!

But as a nod to the "status quo"
Let me just say...

Although this plant was initially discovered for its beneficial properties thousands of years ago, only recently has moringa (sometimes called the Ben oil tree) become known as one of the most impressive herbal supplements to hit the holistic health market. In fact, in 2008 the National Institute of Health called moringa (*moringa oleifera*) the "plant of the year," acknowledging that "perhaps like no other single species, this plant has the potential to help reverse multiple major environmental problems and provide for many unmet human needs." Clearly, moringa benefits are highly touted and deservedly so.

To date, over 1,300 studies, articles and reports have focused on moringa benefits and this plant's healing abilities that are important in parts of the world that are especially susceptible to disease outbreak and nutritional deficiencies. Research shows that just about every part of the moringa plant can be utilized in some way, whether it's to make a potent antioxidant tea or produce an oily substance that lubricates and nourishes the skin. Moringa Oleifera is a fast-growing tree native to South Asia and now found throughout the tropics. Its leaves have been used as part of traditional medicine for centuries, and the Ayurvedic system of medicine associates it with the cure or prevention of about 300 diseases.

Moringa, sometimes described as the "miracle tree," "drumstick tree," or "horseradish tree," has small, rounded leaves that are packed with an incredible amount of nutrition: protein, calcium, beta-carotene, Vitamin C, potassium... you name it, Moringa's got it. No wonder it's been used medicinally (and as a food source) for at least 4,000 years.

The fact that moringa grows rapidly and easily makes it especially appealing for impoverished areas, and it's been used successfully for boosting nutritional intake in Malawi, Senegal, and India for many decades. In these areas, Moringa may be the most nutritious food locally available, and it can be harvested year-round.

Throughout the world, moringa is used for treating such widespread conditions as:

- inflammation-related diseases
- cancer
- diabetes
- anemia
- arthritis and other joint pain, such as rheumatism
- allergies and asthma
- constipation, stomach pains and diarrhea
- epilepsy
- stomach and intestinal ulcers or spasms
- chronic headaches
- heart problems, including high blood pressure
- kidney stones
- fluid retention
- thyroid disorders

- low sex drive
- bacterial, fungal, viral and parasitic infections

Personally, I have grown a moringa tree and I can attest to the fact that it grows like a weed. For those living in third-world countries, it may very well prove to be a valuable source of basic human nutrition.

However, I don't recommend planting one in your backyard for health purposes **unless you understand** that the leaves are very small and it can be a timely and tedious task to harvest them from the stem to eat them. Personally I am fine with that, I enjoy the peacefulness of it, but if it is not for you then you should look into buying your Moringa online!

The leaves are tiny and difficult to harvest and use, so you'll likely find, as many people do, that growing one is more trouble than it seems to be worth.

That being said, there is no denying that Moringa offers an impressive nutritional profile that makes it appealing once it *is* harvested...

8 Reasons Why Moringa Is Being Hailed as a Superfood

1. ### A Rich Nutritional Profile
   Moringa leaves are loaded with vitamins, minerals, essential amino acids, and more. One hundred grams of dry moringa leaf contains:

   9 times the protein of yogurt

   10 times the vitamin A of carrots

   15 times the potassium of bananas

   17 times the calcium of milk

   12 times the vitamin C of oranges

25 times the iron of spinach

2. Antioxidants Galore

Moringa leaves are rich in antioxidants, including vitamin C, beta-carotene, quercetin, and chlorogenic acid. The latter, chlorogenic acid, has been shown to slow cells' absorption of sugar and animal studies have found it to lower blood sugar levels. As noted in the *Asian Pacific Journal of Cancer Prevention*:

> *"The leaves of the* **Moringa oleifera** *tree have been reported to demonstrate antioxidant activity due to its high amount of polyphenols.*
>
> **Moringa oleifera** *extracts of both mature and tender leaves exhibit strong antioxidant activity against free radicals, prevent oxidative damage to major biomolecules, and give significant protection against oxidative damage."*

Further, in a study of women taking 1.5 teaspoons of moringa leaf powder daily for three months, blood levels of antioxidants increased significantly.

3. Balances Hormones and Slows the Effects of Aging

A 2014 study published in the *Journal of Food Science and Technology* tested the effects of moringa (sometimes also called "drumstick") along with amaranth leaves (*Amaranthus tricolor*) on levels of inflammation and oxidative stress in menopausal adult women. Knowing that levels of valuable antioxidant enzymes get affected during the postmenopausal period due to deficiency of "youthful" hormones, including estrogen, researchers wanted to investigate if these superfoods could help slow the effects of aging using natural herbal antioxidants that balance hormones naturally.

Ninety postmenopausal women between the ages of 45–60 years were selected and divided into three groups given various levels of the supplements. Levels of antioxidant status, including serum retinol, serum ascorbic acid, glutathione peroxidase, superoxide dismutase and malondialdehyde were analyzed before and after supplementation, along with fasting blood glucose and haemoglobin levels. Results showed that supplementing with moringa and amaranth caused significant increases in antioxidant status along with significant decreases in markers of oxidative stress.

Better fasting blood glucose control and positive increases in haemoglobin were also found, which led the researchers to conclude that these plants have therapeutic potential for helping to prevent complications due to aging and natural hormonal changes. Moringa benefits the libido as well and might work like a natural birth control compound, according to some studies.

Although it's been used as a natural aphrodisiac to increase sex drive and performance for thousands of years, it seems to help reduce rates of conception. That being said, it can boost the immune system during pregnancy and also increase breast milk production and lactation, according to some studies.

4. **Helps Improve Digestive Health**

Due to its anti-inflammatory properties, moringa has been used in ancient systems of medicine such as Ayurveda to prevent or treat stomach ulcers, liver disease, kidney damage, fungal or yeast infections (such as candida), digestive complaints, and infections.

A common use of moringa oil is helping to boost liver function and therefore detoxifying the body of harmful substances, such as heavy metal toxins. It might also be capable of helping to fight kidney stones, urinary tract infections, constipation, fluid retention/edema and diarrhea.

5. Lower Blood Sugar Levels

As a Diabetic myself I love this! Moringa has anti-diabetic effects, most likely due to so many beneficial plant compounds contained in the leaves, including isothiocyanates. One study found women who took seven grams of moringa leaf powder daily for three months reduced their fasting blood sugar levels by 13.5 percent. Separate research revealed that adding 50 grams of moringa leaves to a meal reduced the rise in blood sugar by 21 percent among diabetic patients. For those of you not living with diabetes let me assure you that those numbers are truly significant.

6. Reduce Inflammation

The isothiocyanates, flavonoids, and phenolic acids in moringa leaves, pods, and seeds also have anti-inflammatory properties. According to the Epoch Times:

"The tree's strong anti-inflammatory action is traditionally used to treat stomach ulcers. Moringa oil (sometimes called Ben oil) has been shown to protect the liver from chronic inflammation. The oil is unique in that, unlike most vegetable oils, moringa resists rancidity.

This quality makes it a good preservative for foods that can spoil quickly. This sweet oil is used for both frying or in a salad dressing. It is also used topically to treat antifungal problems, arthritis, head lice, and is an excellent skin moisturizer."

7. Maintain Healthy Cholesterol Levels

Moringa also has cholesterol-lowering properties, and one animal study found its effects were comparable to those of the widely used cholesterol-lowering drug simvastatin. As noted in the *Journal of Ethnopharmacology*:

> *"Moringa oleifera is used in Thai traditional medicine as cardiotonic. Recent studies demonstrated its hypocholesterolemic effect.*
>
> *... In hypercholesterol-fed rabbits, at 12 weeks of treatment, it significantly lowered the cholesterol levels and reduced the atherosclerotic plaque formation to about 50 and 86%, respectively. These effects were at degrees comparable to those of the drug simvastatin.*
>
> *... The results indicate that this plant possesses truly astounding antioxidant, hypolipidaemic, and antiatherosclerotic activities, and has therapeutic potential for the prevention of cardiovascular diseases."*

8. Protect Against Arsenic Toxicity

The leaves and seeds of moringa may protect against some of the effects of arsenic toxicity, which is especially important in light of news that common staple foods the world over, such as rice, may be contaminated. Contamination of ground water by arsenic has also become a cause of global public health concern, and one study revealed:

"Co-administration of **M. oleifera** *[moringa] seed powder (250 and 500 mg/kg, orally) with arsenic significantly increased the activities of SOD [superoxide dismutase], catalase, and GPx with elevation in reduced GSH level in tissues (liver, kidney, and brain).*

These changes were accompanied by approximately 57%, 64%, and 17% decrease in blood ROS [reactive oxygen species], liver metallothionein (MT), and lipid peroxidation respectively in animal co-administered with **M. oleifera** *and arsenic.*

Another interesting observation has been the reduced uptake of arsenic in soft tissues (55% in blood, 65% in liver, 54% in kidneys, and 34% in brain) following administration of **M. oleifera** *seed powder (particularly at the dose of 500 mg/kg).*

It can thus be concluded from the present study that concomitant administration of **M. oleifera** *seed powder with arsenic could significantly protect both humans and animals from oxidative stress and in reducing tissue arsenic concentration levels. Administration of* **M. oleifera** *seed powder thus could also be beneficial during chelation therapy..."*

From a digestive standpoint, moringa is high in fiber that, as the Epoch Times put it,

"works like a mop in your intestines... to clean up any of that extra grunge left over from a greasy diet."

Also noteworthy are its isothiocyanates, which have anti-bacterial properties that may help to rid your body of H. pylori, a bacteria implicated in gastritis, ulcers, and gastric cancer. Moringa seeds have even been found to work better for water purification than many of the conventional synthetic materials in use today. According to Uppsala University:

"A protein in the seeds binds to impurities causing them to aggregate so that the clusters can be separated from the water. The study... published in the journal **Colloids and Surfaces** *takes a step towards optimization of the water purification process.*

Researchers in Uppsala together with colleagues from Lund as well as Namibia, Botswana, France, and the USA have studied the microscopic structure of aggregates formed with the protein.

The results show that the clusters of material (flocs as they are called) that are produced with the protein are much more tightly packed than those formed with conventional flocculating agents. This is better for water purification as such flocs are more easily separated."

There is speculation that Moringa's ability to attach itself to harmful materials may also happen in the body, making moringa a potential detoxification tool.

How to Use Moringa

If you have access to a moringa tree, you can use the fresh leaves in your meals; they have a flavor similar to a radish. Toss them like a salad, blend them into smoothies, or steam them like spinach. Another option is to use moringa powder, either in supplement form or added to smoothies, soups, and other foods for extra nutrition. Moringa powder has a distinctive "green" flavor, so you may want to start out slowly when adding it to your meals.

You can also use organic, cold-pressed moringa oil (or ben oil), although it's expensive (about 15 times more than olive oil). As mentioned, while I don't necessarily recommend that planting a Moringa tree in your backyard is for everyone as it is a rapid-growing tree can grow to 15 to 30 feet in just a few years, you may want to give the leaves or powder a try if you come across some at your local health food market. In all honesty I really do wish everyone would plant one of these amazing trees in their landscape, if for no other reason than the positive effects that many moringa trees could have on CO_2 in the atmosphere!

As reported by Fox News, this is one plant food that displays not just one or two but *numerous* potential healing powers:

> *"Virtually all parts of the plant are used to treat inflammation, infectious disorders, and various problems of the cardiovascular and digestive organs, while improving liver function and enhancing milk flow in nursing mothers. The uses of moringa are well documented in both the Ayurvedic and Unani systems of traditional medicine, among the most ancient healing systems in the world.*
> *Moringa is rich in a variety of health-enhancing compounds, including moringine, moringinine, the potent antioxidants quercetin, kaempferol, rhamnetin, and various polyphenols. The leaves seem to be getting the most market attention, notably for their use in reducing high blood*

pressure, eliminating water weight, and lowering cholesterol.

Studies show that moringa leaves possess anti-tumor and anti-cancer activities, due in part to a compound called niaziminin. Preliminary experimentation also shows activity against the Epstein-Barr virus. Compounds in the leaf appear to help regulate thyroid function, especially in cases of over-active thyroid. Further research points to anti-viral activity in cases of Herpes simplex 1."

So there you have it. More Moringa information than you can shake a stick at! I truly hope you find it as useful and as informative as I did while I was researching the book!

A Final thought ...

There once was a village chief named Ramasu.
He was known for his wisdom, but he was getting old.

One day a young, ambitious man appeared before
him. "Ramasu, I challenge you to a public contest,"
he said. "I will ask you one question. If you cannot
answer correctly, I will become the new chief."

On the contest day, the whole village showed up
filled with anticipation. The young challenger stepped
forward. "In my hands is a bird. Is it dead or alive?"

The crowd grew silent, knowing the implication.
If Ramasu said "Alive," the young man would
crush the little bird. If he said "Dead," he would
let the bird fly. Either way, Ramasu was trapped.

Ramasu thought for a moment, and then gently
replied, "The life of the bird is in your hands."

Like the living bird in the parable, the life-saving
promise of the Moringa tree is in your hands.

Please act with wisdom.

Throughout this book I have touted the benefits of Moringa and encouraged the reader to grow their own. Then here in the conclusion of the book, I said that growing the tree yourself may not be for everyone. There is no contradiction here, I simply wanted to be as honest about things as possible.

Bottom line?

GROW IT, Eat it, Use it, Share it, and Love it!!!

Be a part of the solution to malnutrition worldwide.

Help plant Moringa trees.

Are you interested in growing your very own Moringa Oleifera tree? Go to Phytonutrient Farms!

If you need seed, you no doubt want to begin with highest quality seeds you can find. That's what we offer at Phytonutrient Farms. To purchase the very best quality, organic non-GMO seeds for all of your growing needs (including Moringa)

Visit:

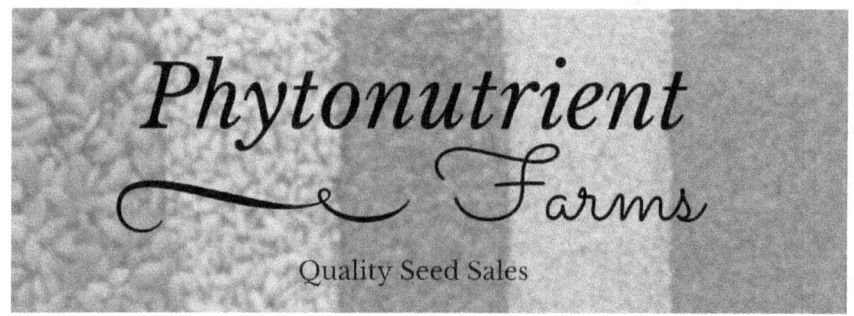

Quality Seed Sales

www.phytonutrientfarms.com

For more and continuing information on Moringa, Phytonutrients, the GMO fight, and much, much more be sure to subscribe to the Phytonutrient Blog with Joe Urbach by visiting:

www.GardeningAustin.com

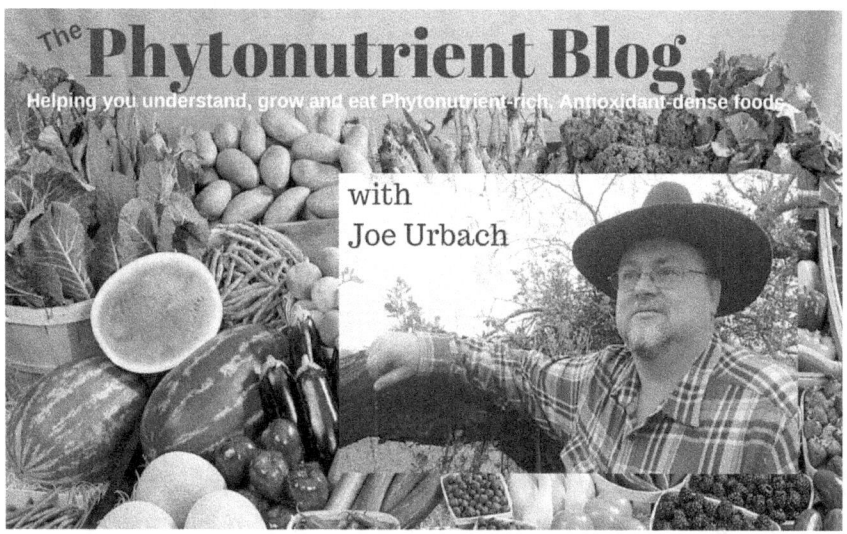

Afterword – The Francis Olaniyi Story

Following is a story that truly impressed me and I wanted to work it into the book in some creative way, I failed to do that so I am just going to include it here. This story is taken off of the website of the organization **Trees For Life** with great appreciation. Please visit and support them at:

http://www.treesforlife.org/

What one young person can do to spread the word about Moringa

Meet Francis O. Olaniyi, a proud member of National Youth Service Corps of Nigeria.

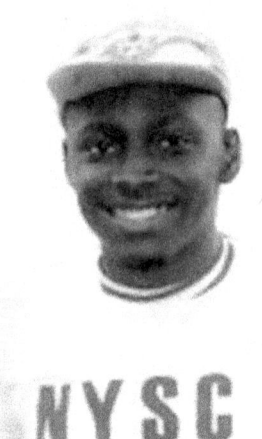

From January of 2012 up till the beginning of June, Trees for Life staff had multiple email exchanges with a young Nigerian named Francis Olaniyi. At that time Francis was half way into a yearlong project of working on MORINGA sensitization throughout Nigeria. It was kicked off in Pil Gani community in Plateau State where there are lots of Moringa trees. His was a year of volunteering through the Nigerian National Youth Service.

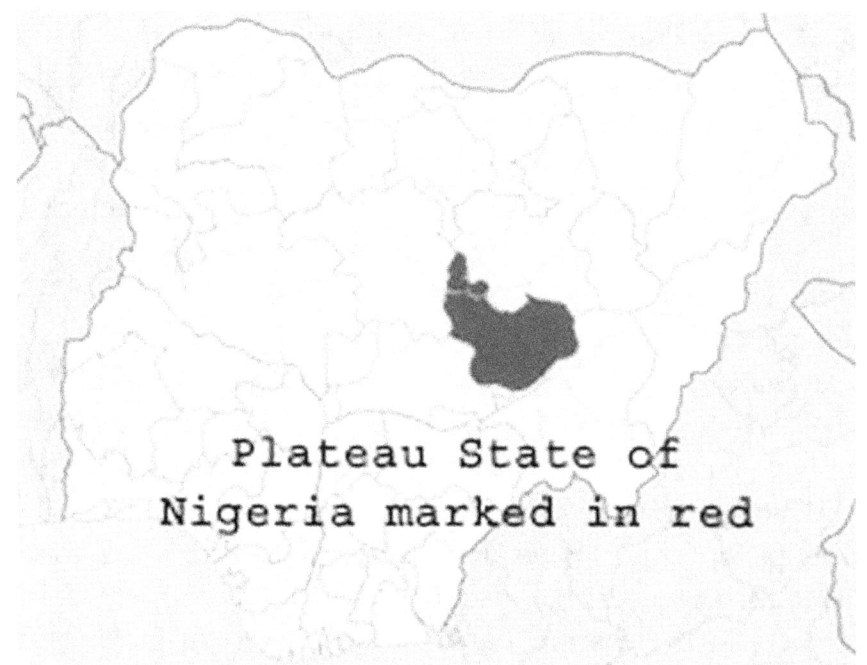

Plateau State of
Nigeria marked in red

Our initial response was to determine in what ways Trees for Life could be helpful to Francis in his plans to spread awareness about this remarkable tree. We learned that Francis was an accounting graduate from Obafemi Awolowo University in South-West Nigeria. "What I love most is touching lives positively, and want to spread the good news of Moringa to as many as possible, educate rural dwellers......curb poverty, reduce malnutrition....and improve material health.

Also, to educate the government, NGOs and others and get them involved in using Moringa to better peoples' lives with a focus on children, youth and women." We couldn't have said it better ourselves!

Francis continues, "Futhermore, I am currently coordinating the MORINGA LOVERS project and working with other volunteers, community heads, farmers, secondary & primary school students and several youth and women's groups." These goals are all a part of his one-year time of service!

To assist Francis, a variety of printed materials were sent to him to use in creating his own translations in the Hausa language. He felt this would further encourage more cultivation, use and commercialisation of Moringa in the rural communities. Three weeks after shipping the materials, Francis confirmed their arrival.

In early June of this year, Francis again wrote to us: "At this juncture, let me say it has been nice knowing "trees for life". As a matter of fact, the people in Langtang North Local government and Plateau State as a whole are much more aware about MORINGA now, especially the need to plant more trees, the need for farmers to cultivate large plantations and the need for the government and the private companies to invest in Moringa. I have facilitated workshops for farmers, who are already making plans to start large cultivations. The media has also helped me in my awareness. Some researchers in the country have shown interest in making more findings on the Moringa to further bring out more facts. I was featured on a national TV program, 'NTA AM Express' on Saturday March 23rd to share with the whole nation and the international community how Moringa can address major health challenges in Africa."

Francis said he has plans, now that he is finished with his National Youth Service Corps year in Plateau State, to move to the southern part of the country, but Moringa awareness continues strongly in his future.

Francis' story is not quite yet over! In July we were told he would be sending two copies of an educational booklet that he had written entitled: MORINGA Lovers – An Adventure of Corper Zogale (Corps Member Moringa – one who educates others about Moringa).

The Moringa Lovers Handbook Authored by Francis O. Olaniyi is shown here.

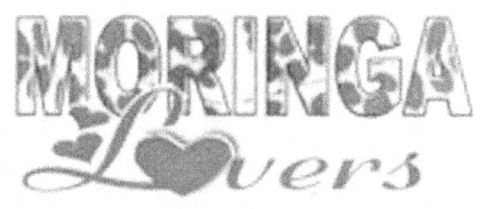

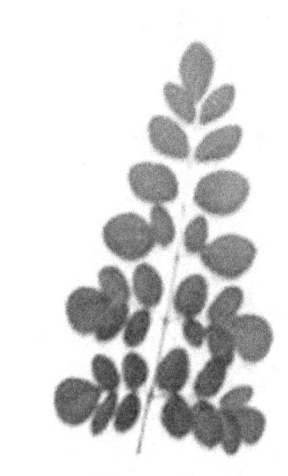

In it, Francis tells how he learned about moringa from his "mum", ended up in the National Youth Service Corps and detailed his many ideas and experiences during his year with the people in Plateau State, Nigeria. Francis closes his story by challenging the reader that "It is never too late to start maximizing the wonderful endowments of Moringa. Help yourself, help your neighbour, help your environment and help the world at large."

We are amazed by all that Francis accomplished during his year of service! A true inspiration to others.

By the way, it is estimated that The efforts of Francis have led to the planting of half a million Moringa trees! Way to go, Francis!

The following are photos taken by Francis of his work with Moringa tree planting.

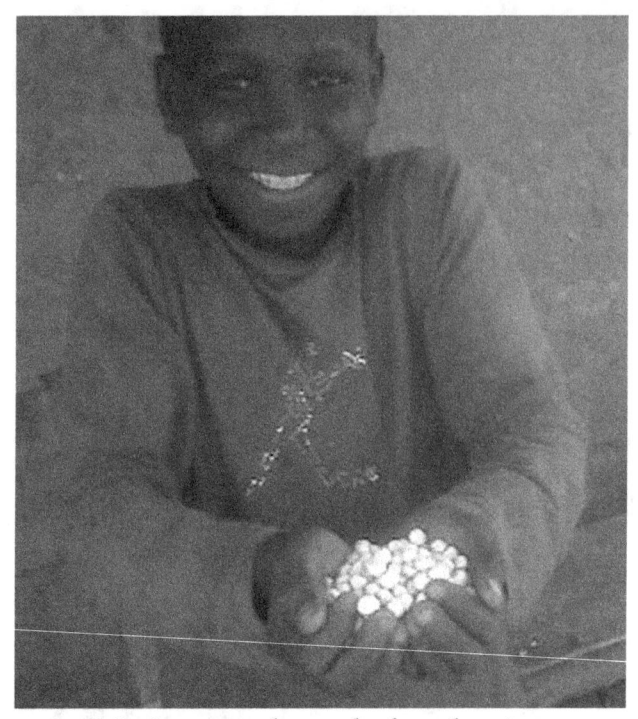

Moringa seeds ready for planting

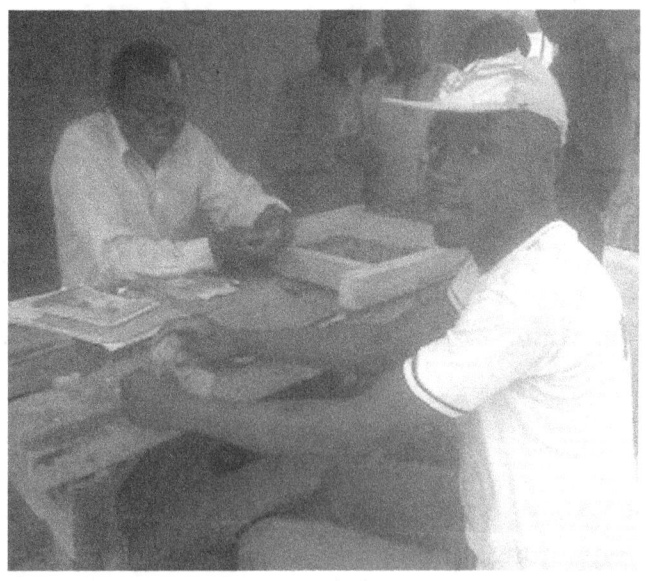

Removing the outer shell of Moringa seeds

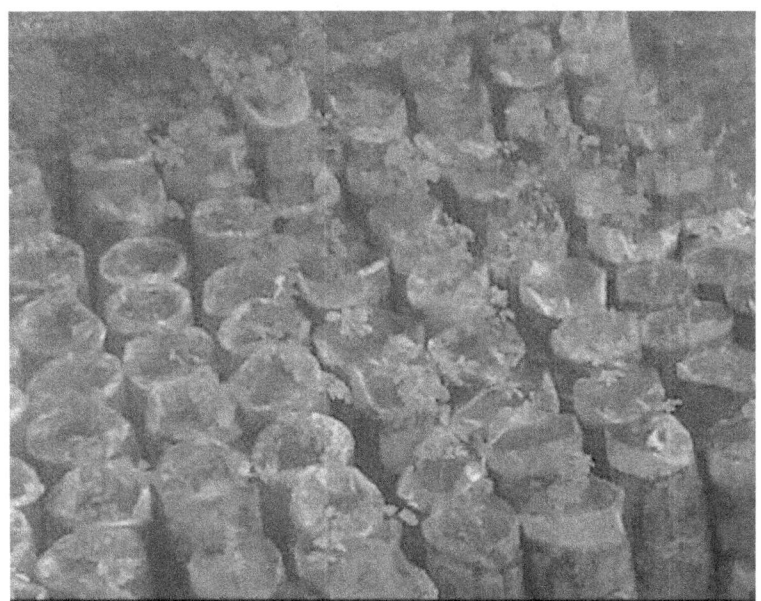

Moringa seedlings after two weeks

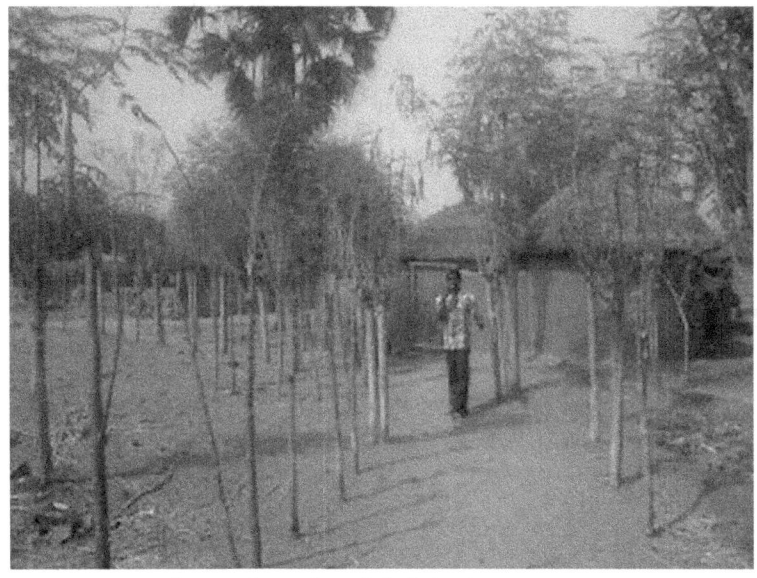

A road path with Moringa trees

Be a part of the solution to malnutrition worldwide.

Help plant Moringa trees.

Are you interested in growing your very own Moringa Oleifera tree? Go to Phytonutrient Farms!

If you need seed, you no doubt want to begin with highest quality seeds you can find. That's what we offer at Phytonutrient Farms. To purchase the very best quality, organic non-GMO seeds for all of your growing needs (including Moringa) Visit:

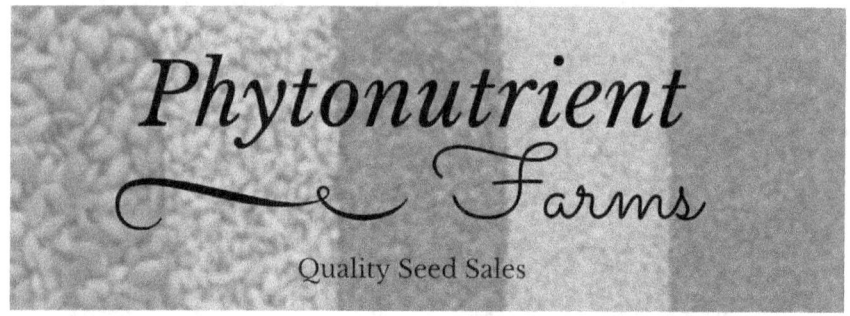

www.phytonutrientfarms.com

For more, and for ongoing information about the benefits of Moringa, or Phytonutrients, or the fight against GMOs and much, much more be sure to subscribe to the Phytonutrient Blog with Joe Urbach by visiting:

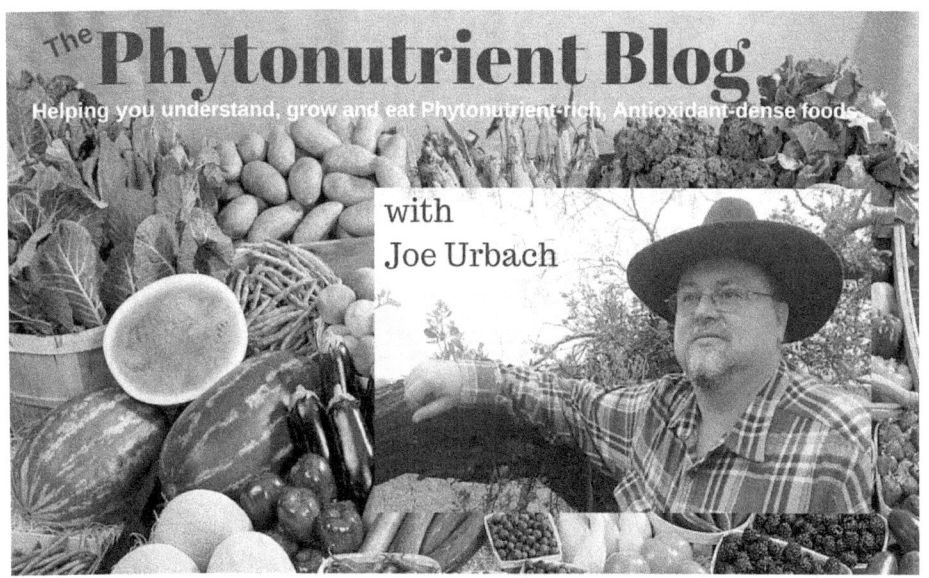

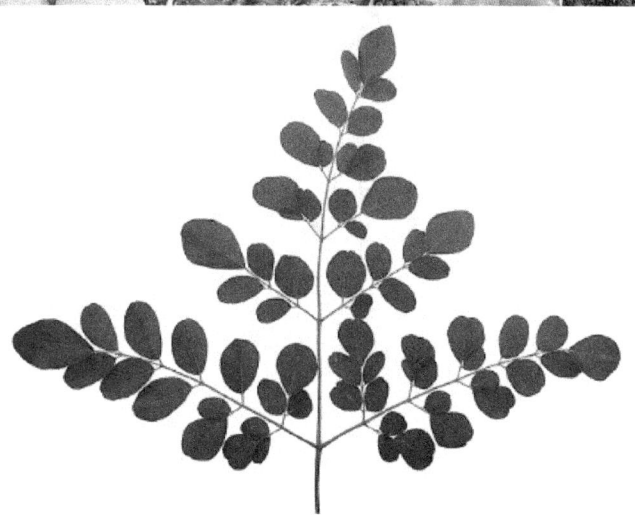